THE *Mediterranean* DIABETES COOKBOOK

AMY RIOLO

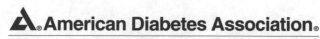

American Diabetes Association.
Cure • Care • Commitment®

Director, Book Publishing, Robert Anthony; *Managing Editor, Book Publishing,* Abe Ogden; *Editor,* Greg Guthrie; *Production Manager,* Melissa Sprott; *Composition,* ADA; *Cover Design,* Vis-à-Vis Creative Concepts; *Food Photography,* Taran Z Studio; *Food Styling,* Lisa Cherkasky; *Printer,* United Graphics, Inc.

Cover Photograph: Caprese-Style Chicken Breasts, page 86.

Printed in the United States of America
5 7 9 10 8 6

ADA titles may be purchased for business or promotional use or for special sales. To purchase more than 50 copies of this book at a discount, or for custom editions of this book with your logo, contact the American Diabetes Association at the address below, at booksales@diabetes.org, or by calling 703-299-2046.

American Diabetes Association
1701 North Beauregard Street
Alexandria, Virginia 22311

DOI: 10.2337/9781580403122

Library of Congress Cataloging-in-Publication Data

Riolo, Amy.
The Mediterranean diabetes cookbook / Amy Riolo.
    p. cm.
Includes bibliographical references and index.
ISBN 978-1-58040-312-2 (alk. paper)
1. Diabetes--Diet therapy. 2. Cookery, Mediterranean. I. Title.
RC662.R515 2010
641.5'6314--dc22

2009045264

In loving memory of my uncle
Sebastian L. Foti,
who, in addition to inspiring me to
travel, study, and cook, shared his
love and knowledge of the Mediterranean with me.

Contents

Foreword

As a nutritionist, I counsel many people with diabetes in choosing foods to help them lower and maintain a healthy blood glucose level and to lead a more healthful lifestyle. In my work, I often find that people are afraid of food. They do not know what to choose, how to choose it, or what is OK and not OK for them to eat. This rings true especially for my clients with diabetes. They don't know what to eat, and just as importantly, they don't know how to enjoy their food. As their blood glucose rises, the sweetness in their lives often diminishes, leaving them feeling distraught and somewhat hopeless. The number one complaint I hear is that they are bored, frustrated, and scared. They feel as though they have little pleasure in the way of food and, as a result, little to look forward to or to enjoy with friends and family. The problem is often compounded by the need to prepare separate meals for themselves.

Food carries such pleasure for each and every one of us, and a person with diabetes is no exception. Not only does our food supply our bodies with essential nutrients, but it is also the very essence by which we form, cultivate, and maintain so many of our important social and familial ties. It is a method by which we nourish and nurture our loved ones and ourselves.

As our lives have become so filled with activities, our food choices have greatly suffered. Many of us find the time to meet our deadlines, watch our favorite television shows, and attend our favorite social and sporting events, yet we don't take the time to prepare our food and enjoy our meals. Taking the time to choose wholesome food and eat well has become a thing of the distant past. In contrast, in the Mediterranean region, these activities are central to a vibrant life, and this book brings us right back to these core values that are so essential for the nourishment of body, mind, and spirit.

People with diabetes must base their meals on quality proteins, whole grains, and legumes; healthful fruits and vegetables; natural and healthful fats; and quality dairy products with the least amount of artificial additives and chemical preservatives. In the *Mediterranean Diabetes Cookbook*, Amy Riolo has expounded on this way of thinking and eating, bringing both pleasure and health back to the table. The recipes are uncomplicated, delicious, and focused on taste, health, and appeal, using traditional ingredients and flavors that make Mediterranean cuisine so popular.

In my practice, I have often noted how changing one's thoughts from fear and discouragement to excitement, anticipation, and enjoyment of food and life can improve well-being. The people of the Mediterranean region enjoy optimal health and longevity due in part to their attitudes and appreciation of food. There, people understand that the spirit in which food is offered and consumed is every bit as important as the food itself. In this cookbook of luscious recipes, you will find healthy foods and living traditions that can easily be incorporated into your own life. With recipes as tasty as these, transitioning to a healthy diet and lifestyle for a person with diabetes becomes pleasurable and exciting.

There is absolutely no deprivation with this fine cookbook. Ms. Riolo teaches us in simple ways how to prepare the freshest food with the finest ingredients. She incorporates such simple delicacies as ripe red tomatoes, eggplant, fresh herbs, extra virgin olive oil, whole grains and legumes indigenous to the region, and tahini, just to name a few.

Seafood, so common to the Mediterranean, is creatively introduced with such mouth-watering recipes as **Tunisian Tuna, Tomato, and Egg Turnovers**; **Poached Sea Bass with Tomatoes and**

Herbs; **Fish Croquettes**; and **French Sole with Mushrooms and Asparagus**.

And just take a look at the celebratory desserts! There you will find great pleasure as you sample the **French Meringue with Rose Cream, Strawberry Mascarpone Parfaits, Yogurt Custard with Figs and Pistachios**, and **Pineapple Tiramisu**.

No longer should any person with diabetes feel forced to choose tasteless packaged, processed, and artificially flavored foods for his or her daily diet. This cookbook changes all of that by relying on traditional foods and ingredients, accompanied by valuable tips and techniques that have been practiced and handed down for centuries in the Mediterranean.

Alana Sugar, CN
www.alanasugar.com

Acknowledgments

I would like to thank my creator for the opportunity to write this book. With each book I write, I realize that recipes are not just formulas written down and exchanged, but a culmination of life's lessons and experience. Everyone who has been a part of my life at one point or another has had a profound effect on my cooking, writing, and teaching style.

I am enormously grateful to Sheilah Kaufman for introducing me to editor Robert Anthony and for her excellent editorial support and friendship. I would also like to thank Robert Anthony, Greg Guthrie, and Abraham Ogden for their excellent editorial and professional guidance and for believing in this book from the beginning. This book would not have been possible without the technical knowledge of nutrition expert Lyn Wheeler, who analyzed every menu and recipe in this book. I truly appreciate the assistance of Paula Jacobson, a great friend and editor. Thanks are also due to Taran Z for her beautiful food photography.

I would like to thank my Nonna, Angela Foti, who taught me that cooking plays an important role in maintaining family traditions. I thank my mother, Faith Riolo, for always encouraging me to cook, and my father, Rick Riolo, for sparking my curiosity in the cuisines and cultures of the world. I thank Yia Yia, Mary Riolo, for introducing me to a world full of Greek flavors, and my grandfather, Vince Riolo, for teaching me not to be afraid to change a recipe.

I would like to thank my husband, Maher El Tanbedawy, for introducing me to the stunningly beautiful and dramatic North African region of the Mediterranean and for willingly taste testing all of my recipes. I am grateful to Ms. Rosa Vilella from Valencia, Spain. Each of the Spanish recipes in this book was inspired by the love and style that she infused in everything she did. Her memory continues to live each time I prepare her recipes.

Thank you to Dr. Norton Fishman, Kathleen Ammalee Rogers, Dr. Beth Tedesco, and Dr. Mary Lee Esty for enabling me to fulfill my dreams. In Egypt, I would like to thank Soad El Tanbedawy, Amira Mohsen, Ahmed Edris, Mohamed Edris, Mahmoud Edris, Mahmoud Fathy el Kady, Ahmed Nubi, Chef Ahmed Hashem, Chef Heggag, Chef Hussein, and Chef Mohamed Abdul Fattah for their support and guidance. In Italy, I would like to thank Liana Mari, Mauro Lesti, Marco and Daniela Greco, Clara and Enrica Iatosti, Signora Grazia, Zia Santina, Angela and Enzo Riolo, and Luigi and Maria Fabbiano for fueling my passion for the pleasures of the palate.

I thank nutritionist Alana Sugar for her insight on the challenges that people with diabetes face today. In addition, I would like to thank every shopkeeper, housewife, taxi driver, chef, fisherman, farmer, and restaurateur who answered my questions and provided me with additional insight.

Introduction

"Che felicità...Tutti a tavola si va."

—Italian Proverb
["What happiness!!! Everyone is going to the table!"]

Eating is a frequently utilized sensory experience. We all look forward to good meals that taste great. Taste is the sense that we actively think about enjoying most often. Unfortunately, for people with diabetes and other chronic diseases, eating is often viewed as a taboo subject, mainly because people need to change their eating habits. From the minute most people are diagnosed with diabetes, they become preoccupied with the foods they will no longer be able to enjoy, instead of thinking about the new foods that they'll be able to experience. The idea of eating healthy meals that fit into a diabetes-friendly lifestyle while their entire family is eating "the regular way" becomes depressing.

My mother was diagnosed with type 2 diabetes when I was a teenager. Her doctor, like many others, gave her a list of foods to avoid. Needless to say, many of her favorite foods were on that list. She was also handed a generic diet that was given to many other women in her situation. What I found interesting, even as a young girl, was that no one ever took into consideration what she enjoyed eating. Her new diet made no mention of foods that were beneficial in maintaining blood glucose levels or that provided valuable vitamins and minerals. Long before I ever thought of a career as a food writer, I made my mother a cookbook that would allow her to eat her favorite foods, while following ADA requirements, and that contained recipes rich in vitamins and minerals. My mother took it into her endocrinologist's office, who agreed that the diet would work. Little by little, I noticed more and more family members being diagnosed with diabetes, including my maternal grandmother and paternal grandfather. Many of us considered genetics to be a major factor. After finishing college, I had the opportunity to travel to southern Italy to meet extended relatives. None of them had any trouble with diabetes and enjoyed full, lush diets, including large, multi-course lunches every day. Even those who owned bakeries were successful in maintaining healthy blood glucose levels. For the next decade, I had the opportunity to travel extensively through the Mediterranean region and found, like many others have, that both the American diet and lifestyle contribute to our growing diabetes epidemic.

The Mediterranean Diabetes Cookbook was written to promote a healthy and pleasurable attitude toward eating and living that Americans could easily adapt to their own lifestyles. I vowed to banish "watered-down" recipes and avoid sugar substitutes. I have included recipes that everyone can love—diabetes or not. Many recipes from the Mediterranean region with which we are already familiar in the U.S. are the fattening, calorie-laden recipes reserved for celebrations and holidays. There is, however, an entire world of delicious and sensible recipes enjoyed by everyone, from models to fishermen, on a daily basis. The recipes in this book are recipes that real people eat during the course of their daily lives. I have purposely included family-style recipes that can be eaten communally—an aspect of utmost importance for both physical and mental health.

1

In the Mediterranean region, people live to eat and they eat to live. From the shores of southern and eastern Europe to those of the coastline of North Africa, food is a source of economic income, artistic creativity, sensory pleasure, and traditional medicine. For this reason, this region's recipes have become some of the world's most beloved, and its inhabitants enjoy unparalleled health, quality of life, and longevity. Both my personal and professional lives are based on, nourished by, and inspired by the countries around the Mediterranean. The hospitality of the people; the beauty of the landscape; the commitment to producing healthy, sustainable foodstuffs; and the priority given to food, family, and friends are what make me call the Mediterranean home, no matter where I happen to physically live.

By taking inspiration from the Mediterranean region, readers will learn to participate in social family activities that are focused on healthful eating instead of unhealthy habits. Growing herbs, fruits, and vegetables; shopping at farmer's markets; planning meals together; making smart grocery choices; and creating new healthful traditions are all attainable goals for people with diabetes and their families and will enable them to make good food choices for healthy living. Many of the activities mentioned in the book emphasize the importance of exercise. Each recipe in the book contains a "Healthy Living Tradition" to encourage readers to make better, more meaningful choices in their diet and lifestyle.

Many people faced with diabetes try to avoid thinking about food, as if food is the enemy that causes illness. *The Mediterranean Diabetes Cookbook* is based on an opposing theory. By focusing on the healthy foods and food-based activities that you love, planning meals ahead of time, and partaking in these delicious recipes with family and friends, you will be healthier and happier.

The recipes have been streamlined into simple, easy-to-follow formats. They can be created with ingredients that are easy to find at supermarkets. Many of these recipes are tried-and-true family recipes that I have been preparing and teaching for years. Other recipes were shared with me by nutritionists, members of the diplomatic community, culinary colleagues, and generous food lovers whom I have met while traveling and living in the Mediterranean region. The recipes are fun to prepare (and make perfect dishes for entertaining), yet are simple enough for beginners and exciting enough for chefs to appreciate. Each recipe contains time-saving tips, concise preparation instructions, and accurate measurements.

The recipe headers contain cultural and historical information pertaining to the country of origin. According to Dr. Brian Wansink, author of *Mindless Eating,* people often value food more and eat less when it is described to them before eating. This extra information makes great conversation. I've found that the novelty of new items and the appeal of faraway places can even encourage finicky children to eat something they're unfamiliar with. It is my goal that *The Mediterranean Diabetes Cookbook* will encourage people to create more family meals and participate in family-centered activities that promote a healthy attitude towards food. I wish you a lifetime of meals. As the Egyptians say, "*Bil hanna wi shefa*! [With pleasure and health!]"

How to Use This Book

This book was created to help people with diabetes make healthful eating and lifestyle decisions, which will bring pleasure to their own lives as well as the lives of their family members. Begin perusing the introductions to each chapter to learn the role of each course in traditional Mediterranean dining. Next, create a time plan and grocery list to try a new recipe. As a cooking instructor, I like to advise reading through each recipe thoroughly at least once before you begin cooking. You'll be amazed at how simple and fun it can be to approach food the Mediterranean way. Enjoy!

Use this book to:

1 Witness how cultures in the region approach meal courses

2 Learn healthy living habits from the tips in each recipe

3 Implement meal planning strategies used by people in the Mediterranean region

4 Look for recipes that include produce which is currently in season in your area

5 Start a Mediterranean Pantry

6 Discover cultural and regional secrets to promoting optimal health

7 Develop enjoyable new habits and traditions for yourself and your family

8 Prepare simple yet impressive meals that everyone will love

9 Create quick, go-to meal plans for busy times

For best results:

1 Make a conscious commitment to eating and living with both pleasure and health in mind

2 Adopt the Mediterranean attitude of taking pride in eating healthful, homemade foods

3 Be willing to experiment with new flavors and ingredient combinations

4 Value freshness and quality of ingredients over quantity

What Is Mediterranean Cuisine?

The term "Mediterranean" is often used to describe cuisine that comes from various countries in the region surrounding the Mediterranean Sea. When most people think of the Mediterranean, however, they think of Italy and Greece and forget about the other countries in southern and eastern Europe as well as North Africa and the Middle East, which share the same shores. Despite the fact that countries like France, Turkey, and Libya share different terrains, climates, and cultures, their proximity to the Mediterranean Sea, years of trade and interaction, and similar attitudes toward cuisine have contributed to create common denominators in the dishes of the region.

Characteristics of Mediterranean Cuisine

1   Wide use of olive oil and citrus juice in cooking.

2   Majority of diet is based on fresh, seasonal, local, and organic produce.

3   Abundance of freshly caught seafood.

4   Small portions of lean meat and poultry are enjoyed.

5   Mealtime is honored as an important ritual in daily life.

6   Beans, nuts, and legumes are important and frequently used staples.

7   Desserts are limited to special occasions.

8   Fresh, homemade food is considered a necessity.

9   Unique herb and spice blends are used to enhance flavors.

10 Walking and other forms of daily physical activity are practiced.

11 Main meals are eaten in the early afternoon; smaller, lighter meals are enjoyed in the evenings.

Achieving the Mediterranean Lifestyle

When we think of the Mediterranean region, we often think of relaxing images of people leading simple lifestyles who have nothing better to do than prepare good food and eat it. It seems like a dream, as if people in that part of the world are living in an alternate reality. When we think of the demands of our own busy lifestyles, which are full of heavy work schedules, numerous activities for our children, social engagements, and time for exercise, it seems impossible to do anything differently from what we are already doing.

What many people fail to realize, however, is that even though the cultures in the Mediterranean focus on healthy eating habits and nutritious food, its people have worked very hard to maintain those traditions by demanding that good nutrition and healthy lifestyles be a basic right, not a luxury. Even today, with working moms, demanding jobs, traffic, and other constraints, good food and healthy living still prevail. People are constantly adjusting their schedules and personal habits and customs to make sure that they lead healthy lives. By following the lead of the people in this region, Americans will be able to live with both pleasure and health.

Remember that it is difficult to make changes all at once. After reading this section, begin by making and sticking to one change per week or month. Over time, you will find that the new and different activities are fun, beneficial, and worth the effort.

Here are some tips that people in the Mediterranean region use to maintain their healthy lifestyles.

1. Analyze your situation
- Make a list of budget and time concerns in terms of diet and food preparation.
- List health, personal, and family goals for nutrition and lifestyle.
- With your list of desired outcomes in hand, look at a work schedule that also contains family events and socializing.
- Find "pockets" of time to plan meals, grocery shop, and prepare meals.

2. Organize your time
- Decide which pockets of time you will use to prepare food.
- Make healthy meals in advance and refrigerate or freeze them for times when you can't cook.
- Use socializing time as cooking, shopping, or prep time—invite friends and family over for a healthy meal or picnic.
- Meet at each other's homes and prepare food together.
- Delegate food shopping and prepping tasks to friends and family.
- Make food shopping and farmer's markets an activity to be enjoyed with others.

3. Develop a Mediterranean Pantry
- Read "Starting a Mediterranean Pantry" (on p. 13) for tips.
- Use this book and your pantry for inspiration.

4. Plan meals wisely
- Read the "Mediterranean Meal Planner" (on p. 8) for tips.
- Before you go to sleep each night, take some time to decide what you will eat the following day.
- Make sure you have the necessary ingredients.
- If you work outside of the home, plan on making lunch in advance.
- Bring healthful snacks with you wherever you go to avoid eating junk food.
- Save time and money by being your own personal chef!

5. Breakfast
- If your mornings are hurried, keep plenty of low-fat yogurt, cereal, soynuts, part-skim cheeses, low-fat cereal bars, and fresh fruit on hand.
- Make sure that you start your day with the proper nutrients, and don't skip meals.

6. Lunch
- One of the easiest ways to make lunch is to bring leftovers from the previous night's meal. If the nightly meal was wholesome and healthy, you don't have to think about making something separate for lunch. Try making extra at dinner for this purpose.
- If you don't like the idea of eating the same thing two days in a row, freeze large batches of soups and stews in individual portions and defrost them daily to have for lunch.
- Pack salads in individual serving-size containers with dressings on the side to bring to work with soups and stews.
- For days when you can't bring lunch, keep your own homemade "menu" of tasty and healthful lunch items from nearby stores or cafes.

7. Dinner

- Plan weekday dinners on the weekend beforehand.
- Use time over the weekend to begin prepping and preparing meals to cut down on time spent preparing meals after work.
- Choose dishes that are quick, satisfying, and healthful to make during the week.

8. Special Occasions

This is your chance to really get creative and have fun!

- Enjoy the process of creating a delicious seasonal menu for family and friends.
- Make breads and baked goods up to a month in advance and store them in the freezer.
- Indulge in preparing recipes that you normally do not have the time to make.
- Periodically, make your favorite special-occasion meals for everyday dining.

9. Potlucks and Parties

- Use this opportunity to contribute healthful and satisfying dishes.
- Bring a dish that you enjoy and know is nutritionally balanced.

10. Exercise

Exercise is an extremely important factor in the Mediterranean lifestyle, and it keeps people healthy. Nightly walks with family and friends, more walking due to limited parking, and the abundance of stairs promote an active lifestyle all over the region. In the U.S., we definitely need to be more creative in order to achieve healthy weights. We need 30–60 minutes of exercise most days to compensate for our sedentary lifestyle. Ways to incorporate exercise are to:

- play a team sport
- garden
- take the stairs and walk whenever possible
- take walks after meals
- sign up for exercise and/or dance classes
- meet friends and relatives at parks, gyms, sports meets, or lessons, rather than at restaurants
- invite people to walk and window shop while catching up instead of sitting down and talking
- cook your own meals! Shopping for produce at markets, going grocery shopping, preparing food, and cooking are great ways to burn additional calories.

The Mediterranean Lifestyle and Your Diabetes Meal Plan

Maintaining your blood glucose levels is the goal of diabetes management, and the Mediterranean lifestyle can help you achieve this. Following such a diet may help lower blood glucose levels, reduce the risk of heart disease, and delay or prevent the need for medications to treat diabetes. The way people traditionally eat in the Mediterranean is naturally low in saturated fat, is high in the healthier unsaturated fats, and contains a lot of nuts, whole grains, fruits, and vegetables. The focus on using extra-virgin olive oil and eating high-fiber foods helps keep people healthy. In fact, a large-scale study concluded in 2009 offers some evidence that eating a Mediterranean diet was actually better for people with diabetes than following a regular low-fat diet.

Here's why.

All people get their life-giving energy from the food they eat. Food is made up of fat, protein, carbohydrate, and vitamins and minerals. When you eat, your body converts these nutrients into glucose, which then enters your bloodstream. The cells in your body use this blood glucose for energy. While all nutrients affect the amount of glucose that enters your bloodstream, carbohydrate has the biggest impact. Simply put, more carbohydrate equals more glucose in the bloodstream.

Once glucose enters your bloodstream, insulin helps your body absorb this glucose for energy. In a way, insulin acts as a key that opens the door to your body's cells, letting the glucose in. If you have diabetes, you either don't make enough insulin (impaired glucose tolerance) or your insulin doesn't work as well as it once did (insulin resistance). This means not enough glucose is used for energy and too much glucose is left in your bloodstream. Over the years, these high blood glucose levels can lead to long-term complications of diabetes, including heart disease, eye problems, nerve damage, and kidney trouble.

This diabetes situation is compounded by the typical American lifestyle. Americans don't get enough physical activity, and they eat diets filled with fatty foods and not enough fruits and vegetables. People who do not get physical activity can gain weight. Excess weight can make insulin resistance worse, and it puts a burden on an already taxed cardiovascular system. A diet of fatty foods leads to even more weight gain and clogged arteries. This cycle can be disastrous to a person's health.

A Mediterranean lifestyle focuses on healthier meals and more physical activity. Eating fewer processed high-fat foods and getting more whole grains, fruits, and vegetables in the diet reduces the risk of weight gain. It may even lead to weight loss. When people with diabetes lose weight, insulin resistance is often reduced, making insulin and medications work better. There's an extra reward in trying out these dishes, too. The food tastes great!

Make Meals Fit with Nutrition Info

At the end of each recipe, there is a lot of valuable information, including the number of servings per recipe, serving size, exchanges/choices, and nutrition information, so you know exactly what you're putting on your table. Often, it can be difficult figuring out exactly how many carbohydrates or how much protein you'll get out of a homemade dish, which is where this information comes in handy.

Exchanges/choices are a meal-planning tool for people with diabetes. The best way to learn more about them is to meet with your registered dietitian. If you want to use the exchanges/choices to help manage your blood glucose levels, you should purchase a copy of *Choose Your Foods: Exchange Lists for Diabetes* from the American Diabetes Association at http://store.diabetes.org.

Number of servings and **serving size** indicate how many people a recipe will feed and what size a reasonable portion will be. Because portion control is an essential part of diabetes meal planning, this information is invaluable.

The **nutrition information** is just like what you'd find on a package of food in your grocery store: calories, fat, total carbohydrate, protein, etc. Always remember that this information is based on a single serving of that specific recipe, so if you don't follow the serving size information these numbers will not match what you eat. Also, be aware that the nutrition information is based on generic products, so while that information may be pretty close to the nutrition value of the food you prepare, it won't be exact. There are great online resources for learning more about reading food labels. An excellent book that covers this topic is *What Do I Eat Now*, by Patti Geil and Tami Ross, published by the American Diabetes Association.

Mediterranean Meal Planner

"What Grows Together Goes Together"

When planning a Mediterranean menu, it's important to consider the season, region, occasion, and personal traditions. When I develop new menus, I often start with a list of fruits and vegetables that are in season. I choose the ones that my guests and I like, as well as what I may have on hand. Next, I pick a region as a theme and use recipes from there. Considering the occasion means that I think about how much time I will have to prepare something and whether it needs to look extra special for a holiday. Then, I like to incorporate important traditions. For New Year's, lentils must be on the menu; for certain holidays, cookies; and for picnics, lemonade, and so forth.

Textures are the final thing I consider when making a meal. Throughout the Mediterranean region you will find:

1. both cooked and raw vegetables at the same meal

2. at least one of the dishes will have a cream, sauce, stew, or glaze aspect
3. crunchy nuts and crispy fried onions as common garnishes

Each of the following seasonal menus is divided into categories for easy planning and for fitting Mediterranean culinary culture into the American lifestyle. Refer to these menus for planning and inspiration. For additional ideas, please see "Achieving the Mediterranean Lifestyle" (p. 4).

Seasonal Menu Categories

Elegant Mediterranean Evening
Make-Ahead Mediterranean Meal
Easy Mediterranean Entertaining
Sunday Mediterranean Brunch
Mediterranean Spa Meal
Vegetarian Mediterranean Dining
Express Mediterranean Dinner
Mediterranean Holiday

Spring

Elegant Mediterranean Evening
Bruschetta with Artichoke Purée and Roasted Red Peppers (p. 27)
Corsican Prawns with Chickpea Cream (p. 38)
Orange, Asparagus, and Avocado Salad (p. 168)
Raspberry and Lemon Sorbet (p. 219)

Make-Ahead Mediterranean Meal
Escarole and Meatball Soup (p. 64)
Baby Artichokes with Herb Sauce (p. 150)
Mozzarella, Tomato, and Chickpea Salad (p. 190)
Lemony Rice Pudding (p. 206)

Easy Mediterranean Entertaining
Roman Spaghetti with Artichokes, Mint, and Garlic (p. 74)
Sicilian-Style Tuna Steaks (p. 118)
Cucumber, String Bean, and Olive Tapenade Salad (p. 186)
Peaches in Basil-Yogurt Cream (p. 226)

Mediterranean Spa Dinner
Orzo with Lemon, Artichokes, and Asparagus (p. 69)
Salmon with Pea Purée (p. 121)
Mixed Herb Plate (p. 31)
Strawberry Mascarpone Parfaits (p. 204)

Sunday Mediterranean Brunch
Cilantro Pancakes (p. 23)
Spicy Israeli Tomato Spread (p. 33)
Tunisian Tuna, Tomato, and Egg Turnovers (p. 44)
Anise Biscuits (p. 195)
Date, Almond, and Sesame Balls (p. 211)
Sour Cherry Lemonade (p. 239)

Vegetarian Mediterranean Dining
Traditional Chickpea and Tahini Purée (p. 41)
Yogurt and Potato Soup (p. 63)
Bean, Lentil, and Spinach Skillet (p. 164)
Corn, Tomato, Pea, and Dill Salad (p. 185)
French Meringue with Rose Cream (p. 221)

Express Mediterranean Dinner
Veal Scaloppini with Eggplant Veloutè (p. 111)
Sicilian Salad with Potatoes (p. 184)
Almond Milk Cooler (p. 234)

Mediterranean Holiday
Stuffed Vine Leaves (p. 34)
Cucumber, Yogurt, and Dill Salad (p. 22)
Beef and Vegetable Stew (p. 141)
Mint Tea (p. 240)

Summer

Elegant Mediterranean Dinner
Rosemary Focaccia (p. 260)
White Gazpacho Mocktails (p. 58)
Stuffed Chicken Breasts with Cucumber Cream (p. 100)
Moroccan Salad Trio (p. 188)
Melon, Plum, and Nectarine Soup (p. 224)

Make-Ahead Mediterranean Meal
Cool Carrot Purée with Bell Pepper Sticks (p. 20)
Lebanese Bulgur, Tomato, and Cucumber Salad (p. 177)
Chicken, Tomato, and Pepper Stew (p. 137)
Fruit-Filled Phyllo Snake (p. 214)

Easy Mediterranean Entertaining
Spanish Gazpacho Soup Shooters (p. 57)
Greek Chicken Souvlaki (p. 85)
Grilled Italian Vegetables (p. 163)
Shepherd's Salad (p. 181)
Watermelon and Rose Water Granita (p. 218)

Sunday Mediterranean Brunch
Eggplant with Yogurt, Tahini, and Pine Nuts (p. 147)
Circassian Chicken and Lettuce (p. 89)
Nectarines with Mint Sugar (p. 225)
Fig and Fromage D'Affinois Crostini (p. 223)
Orange Blossom and Mint Infused Orange Juice (p. 237)

Express Mediterranean Dinner
Mixed Pepper Medley (p. 161)
Caprese-Style Chicken Breasts (p. 86)
Romaine, Spinach, and Radicchio Salad (p. 172)
Peaches in Basil-Yogurt Cream (p. 226)

Mediterranean Spa Dinner
Celery Purée with Carrot Sticks (p. 22)
Marinated Italian Eggplants (p. 29)
Roasted Cod with Tomatoes, Zucchini, and Olives (p. 116)
Espresso Granita (p. 217)

Vegetarian Mediterranean Dining
Saffron Couscous (p. 76)
Majorcan Vegetable Stew (p. 136)
Carrot, Date, and Orange Salad (p. 176)
Moroccan Tangerine Sorbet (p. 220)
Mint Tea (p. 240)

Mediterranean Holiday
Eggplant Caviar (p. 24)
Chicken Fattah (p. 98)
Rice and Herb Stuffed Tomatoes (p. 68)
Rose and Mint Infused Fruit Salad (p. 230)

Fall

Elegant Mediterranean Dining
Traditional Minestrone (p. 61)
Veal Scaloppini with Roasted Red Peppers and Arugula (p. 108)
Fresh Figs with Raspberry Purée (p. 229)
Classic Italian Espresso (p. 247)

Mediterranean Holiday
Italian Asparagus Soup (p. 50)
Southern French-Style Herb-Roasted Turkey (p. 106)
Spice-Dusted Sweet Potatoes (p. 153)
Warm Goat Cheese Salad (p. 173)
Baked Egyptian Pumpkin Pudding (p. 205)
Anise Tea (p. 241)

Easy Mediterranean Entertaining
Eggplant Caviar (p. 24)
Couscous with Tomatoes, Black Beans, and Herbs (p. 77)
Chicken Breasts with Kumquats (p. 99)
Pineapple Tiramisu (p. 203)
Mint Tea (p. 240)

Sunday Mediterranean Brunch
Rose Tea (p. 242)
Spinach-Stuffed Bread Triangles (p. 264)
Spanish Potato Omelet (p. 26)
Stewed Cannellini Beans with Tomatoes and Sage (p. 159)
Poached Apples in Rose Tea (p. 227)
Tuscan Cantucci Cookies (p. 199)

Mediterranean Spa Meal
Red Lentil Purée (p. 39)
Eggplant and Chickpea Stew (p. 134)
Carrot, Date, and Orange Salad (p. 176)
Ginger Tea (p. 243)

Express Mediterranean Dinner
Dijon-Glazed Chicken Breasts with Zucchini
   (p. 87)
Herb and Olive Oil Mashed Potatoes (p. 155)
Pear and Radicchio Salad with Pistachios (p. 170)
Grapes with Goat Cheese and Almonds (p. 222)
Turkish Coffee with Cardamom (p. 249)

Vegetarian Mediterranean Dining
Saffron Rice with Almonds and Raisins (p. 66)
Spicy Tunisian Chickpea Stew (p. 59)
Cucumber, Yogurt, and Dill Salad (p. 32)
Baked Egyptian Pumpkin Pudding (p. 205)
Turkish Tea (p. 245)

Make-Ahead Mediterranean Meal
Arborio Rice Salad with Vegetables (p. 65)
Chicken Thighs with Tomato-Tarragon Sauce
   (p. 96)
Orange and Fennel Salad (p. 169)
Calabrian Sesame Cookies (p. 198)

Winter

Elegant Mediterranean Dinner
Valencian Seafood Paella (p. 130)
Orange and Fennel Salad (p. 169)
Milk and Rose Water Pudding (p. 207)
Egyptian Cinnamon Tea (p. 246)

Make-Ahead Mediterranean Meal
Roasted Eggplant Purée (p. 40)
Moroccan Harira Soup (p. 53)
Roasted Veal with Root Vegetables (p. 110)
Sweet Couscous (p. 208)

Express Mediterranean Dinner
White Bean and Tomato Soup (p. 55)
Turbot with Watercress and Zucchini (p. 127)
Red Cabbage Salad (p. 171)

Mediterranean Spa Meal
North African Chickpea Soup (p. 54)
Poached Sea Bass with Tomatoes and Herbs
   (p. 117)
Moroccan Salad Trio (p. 188)
Yogurt Custard with Figs and Pistachios (p. 210)

Easy Mediterranean Holiday Entertaining
Cauliflower and Broccoli Purée (p. 21)
White Bean and Tomato Soup (p. 55)
French Roasted Chicken with Green Beans
   (p. 88)
Warm Goat Cheese Salad (p. 173)
Apple, Date, and Raisin Phyllo Strudel (p. 212)
Classic Italian Espresso (p. 247)

Sunday Mediterranean Brunch
Bicerin (p. 248)
Italian Sponge Cake (p. 202)
Fava Bean Purée (p. 36)
Potato-Artichoke Torte (p. 152)

Vegetarian Mediterranean Dining
Lentils and Rice (p. 131)
Stewed Okra and Tomatoes (p. 156)
Egyptian Country Salad (p. 178)
Sweet Vermicelli with Strawberries (p. 216)

Where-to-Buy Guide

Adriana's Caravan
www.adrianascaravan.com
Spices, including baharat, dried lemon, dried rosebuds, fenugreek, saffron, sumac, and zataar. Also, bulgur, couscous, date molasses, fava beans, orange blossom water, pomegranate molasses, rose water, spice grinders, and tahini.

Diamond Organics
1-888-ORGANIC
www.diamondorganics.com
Organic produce, breads, pantry items, seafood, and dairy items.

Kalustyan's
1-212-685-3451
www.kalustyans.com
Arabic coffee (plain or with cardamom), Arabic coffee cups, Arabic coffee pots, bulgur, Ceylon tea, chickpea flour, couscous, dried rose petals, fava beans, fenugreek, grape leaves, grenadine, hulled grain (sold as frik), lavash and pita bread, orange blossom water, rice flour, rose water, tahini, saffron, sesame seeds, sumac, and zataar.

Melissa's/World Variety Produce, Inc.
1-800-588-0151
www.melissas.com
Fresh, seasonal fruits, vegetables, herbs, and spices.

Sur La Table
1-866-328-5412
www.surlatable.com
Cookware, bakeware, specialty foods, and cutlery.

Whole Foods
www.wholefoods.com
Organic and conventional produce, including agave nectar, whole-wheat pastry flour, white whole-wheat flour, grey sea salt, cheeses, seafood, meat, poultry, coffee, tea, breads, and wellness products.

Zabar's
1-212-787-2000
www.zabars.com
Olive oils, spices, teas, fruits, nuts, and cheeses.

Starting a Mediterranean Pantry

Why Does It Matter?

The idea of a pantry, as old fashioned as it may seem, plays an important role in today's busy world, just like it did in antiquity. In the olden days, a pantry was necessary to preserve foods that were not in season and, therefore, not available. Housewives would pickle and preserve seasonal fruits and vegetables with each new crop. During the winter months, they would have the ingredients on hand for nourishment. Grains, spices, teas, and ingredients that could only be found in towns were stored up by villagers between visits, which may have occurred only a few times a year.

In the modern world, many of us live a short distance from some kind of grocery store or supermarket, so why, you may ask, is it necessary to stock a pantry?

The truth of the matter is that a well-stocked pantry can save you time, money, and stress and encourage you to eat healthfully. With a pantry already in place, you can whip up many of the delicious recipes in this book in just minutes. Weekly grocery shopping trips will be faster because you'll only have to shop for fresh ingredients. You will also save yourself a lot of aggravation when you have all of the basics that you need to cook a meal on hand. Equipped with an arsenal of healthful dry goods, you'll be less apt to order or eat out—saving yourself money and calories.

Tips for Keeping a Well-Stocked Pantry

1. *Dedicate an area—no matter how small—to house the ingredients called for in this list.*

2. *Keep a magnetic grocery list on the door and write down each item that is running low.*

3. *Look for pantry items that are on sale and in bulk quantities to save money.*

Items to Stock Your Pantry

The following items are categorized by where they are found in grocery stores.

Baking

Active dry yeast
Agave nectar
Almond extract
Baking powder
Baking soda
Cornstarch
Flour, all-purpose, unbleached
Flour, bread
Flour, chickpea
Flour, whole-wheat pastry
Flour, whole-wheat white
Grey sea salt
Kosher salt
Natural sugar
Pumpkin purée
Sugar
Unsweetened cocoa powder
Vanilla extract

Beans and Legumes

Black beans, canned, reduced-sodium
Cannellini beans, canned, low-sodium
Chickpeas, no-salt-added, canned or dried
Lentils, brown

Herbs (Dried)

Basil
Lavender
Marjoram
Oregano
Rosemary
Sage
Tarragon
Thyme

Italian Specialty

Anchovy fillets, in olive oil
Artichoke hearts, canned
Bread crumbs, plain
Capers, packed in water
Espresso coffee
Ladyfingers
Roasted red peppers, jar
Olives, green, black, Kalamata, Niçoise, and Gaeta
Tomatoes, low-sodium, diced, canned, and fire-roasted
Tomato purée
Tomato paste
Tuna, canned, packed in water

Miscellaneous

Dates
Dijon mustard
Garlic
Granola, low-fat, almond
Honey
Pineapple, canned, crushed, with juice

Nuts and Dried Fruit

Almonds, blanched
Chestnuts, jar, whole, roasted or steamed
Pine nuts
Pistachios, shelled
Raisins

Oils and Vinegars

Canola oil
Corn or vegetable oil, expeller pressed
Nonstick cooking spray
Olive oil, extra-virgin
Vinegar, apple cider
Vinegar, balsamic
Vinegar, white, distilled

Pasta and Grains

Bulgur wheat
Cornmeal
Couscous
Orzo
Polenta
Penne rigate
Rice, Arborio
Rice, basmati
Rice, medium-grain
Spaghetti

Spices

Allspice
Anise seeds
Caraway seeds
Cayenne pepper
Chili powder
Cinnamon and cinnamon sticks
Coriander
Cloves, whole and ground
Crushed dried red chili flakes
Cumin
Fennel seeds
Ginger, dried and ground
Green cardamom, ground and pods
Kosher or sea salt
Mint, dried
Nutmeg
Juniper berries
Paprika
Peppercorns
Saffron
Sumac
Seafood seasoning
Turmeric

Stocks

Chicken stock, reduced-sodium
Vegetable stock, reduced-sodium

Items for the Fridge

Carrots
Celery
Eggs
Fresh seasonal produce
Herbs, fresh
Lemons
Lettuces, assorted
Milk, skim
Onions
Parmesan, Romano, mozzarella, feta, and goat
    cheeses
Potatoes
Shallots
Sweet potatoes
Walnuts, shelled
Yogurt, plain, fat-free

Items for the Freezer

Chicken breasts, boneless, skinless
Fish fillets
Phyllo dough
Vegetables, frozen

Specialty Pantry Items

See the Where-to-Buy Guide for purchasing information.

Dried hibiscus flowers

Dried hibiscus petals are stemmed to make a healthy and delicious tisane in Egypt as well as in African and Caribbean countries.

Dried organic rosebuds

Dried organic rosebuds are used to make teas and add a unique floral component to Middle Eastern dishes.

Egyptian rice or other short-grain rice

Sometimes called Calrose rice, Egyptian rice is a uniquely shaped medium-grain rice, which is a close cousin to Italian Arborio rice. Arborio rice or another medium-grain rice may be substituted, if necessary.

Fava beans (canned, cooked, broad variety)

Large, brown, cooked fava beans are often referred to as broad beans and are known to be one of the world's oldest crops.

Loose-leaf black tea

Look for Darjeeling tea for high-quality taste.

Orange blossom water

Distilled water made from pressed orange blossom petals; used in sweets and salad dressings.

Pomegranate molasses

A rich, tangy molasses made from reduced pomegranate juice; used to flavor dressings, sauces, and marinades.

Preserved lemons

A North African specialty. Lemons are pickled, mixed with various spices, and preserved; they are eaten alone as a condiment or added to soups and stews.

Preserved vine leaves (jar or vacuum-sealed package)

Preserved leaves from grape vines. Many Middle Eastern and Mediterranean grocers stock fresh leaves from California in the spring. Otherwise, use jarred or canned leaves.

Red lentils

Popular in the eastern Mediterranean, they are nutritious, quick cooking, and require no soaking.

Semolina

A yellow flour made from hard wheat. Most frequently used in making sweets and breads, it comes from the layer of wheat that is between the bran and innermost part.

Sesame seeds

These seeds are rich in niacin, phosphorus, and protein. They are inexpensive and can be purchased in large quantities at Mediterranean markets.

Rose water

Water made from distilled organic rose oil; used to flavor syrups, pastries, and breads.

Tahini sauce

A paste-like sauce made from the oil from pressed sesame seeds.

Tamarind syrup

A concentrated, cooked syrup made from tamarind juice.

Turkish coffee

Coarsely ground Arabica coffee that is brewed in a traditional pot on the stovetop and served unfiltered.

Vermicelli

A form of thinly shaped broken pasta used in soups, sweets, and pasta dishes.

Za'taar

A variety of thyme native to the Middle East. It can be used in breads, meat, poultry, soups, and stews. It is known in Arabic as *za'taar*. There is also spice mix that includes wild thyme; it is referred to as *za'taar* in Arabic as well.

Small Plates

Cool Carrot Purée with Bell Pepper Sticks 20
Cauliflower and Broccoli Purée 21
Celery Purée with Carrot Sticks 22
Cilantro Pancakes 23
Eggplant Caviar 24
Spinach Flan 25
Spanish Potato Omelet 26
Bruschetta with Artichoke Purée and Roasted Red Peppers 27
Eggplant Croquettes 28
Marinated Italian Eggplants 29
Carrots with Garlic and Yogurt 30
Mixed Herb Plate 31
Cucumber, Yogurt, and Dill Salad 32
Spicy Israeli Tomato Spread 33
Stuffed Vine Leaves 34
Fava Bean Purée 36
Fish Croquettes 37
Corsican Prawns with Chickpea Cream 38
Red Lentil Purée 39
Roasted Eggplant Purée 40
Traditional Chickpea and Tahini Purée 41
Eggplant, Tomato, and Shallot Baby Calzones 42
Tunisian Tuna, Tomato, and Egg Turnovers 44

Appetizers, Dips, and Purées

Across the Mediterranean region, appetizers are the gateway to fabulous multi-course menus that are full of local specialties. Unlike American appetizers, in which a few items are served in large portions, Mediterranean-style appetizers usually consist of many small plates, which offer great variety and healthful ingredients. In the countries surrounding the Mediterranean, appetizers are typically not included in daily meals in the home, but are beloved starters in restaurants, cafes, and taverns.

In many countries around the region, restaurants serve such complex and satisfying small plates before meals that they could provide a full meal on their own. In some countries, however, appetizers are free when ordered with entrées. For this reason, they are not to eaten by themselves, unless they are offered between meals or as an admittedly meager supper.

There are five distinctively different philosophies regarding small plates around the Mediterranean that are determined by country or region of origin. France, Spain, Italy, the eastern Mediterranean, and North Africa all have their own appetizer customs and cultures, which set the tone for the way a meal should be started. Fresh, warm bread and olives are offered with starters throughout the Mediterranean.

In France, appetizers are seen as a way to showcase a chef's creativity and set the culinary standards for the rest of the meal. In a traditional meal, classical French culinary techniques and standards are evident from the very beginning. Haute cuisine chefs use highly stylized aesthetics to create dazzling bite-size appetizers, which signal that the meal will be a treat for both the eyes and the palate. Mini versions of appetizers are sometimes served in a pre-appetizer course commonly referred to as *amuse bouches* or "mouth amusers."

Cool Carrot Purée with Bell Pepper Sticks (p. 20), *Cauliflower and Broccoli Purée* (p. 21), *Celery Purée with Carrot Sticks* (p. 22), *Cilantro Pancakes* (p. 23), *Eggplant Caviar* (p. 24), and *Spinach Flan* (p. 25) are just a few of the wonderful appetizers that French cuisine has to offer.

Spaniards are lucky to enjoy the wonderful culinary culture of *tapas*—a tradition in which people go out at night and enjoy delicious small plates in restaurants. People congregate with friends, often enjoying one or two dishes from each restaurant. When they've finished at one establishment, they walk to another one nearby, sampling the flavors and atmosphere of each until they're satisfied. Small Spanish plates typically consist of vegetable, fish, and cheese-based dishes. *Tapas* hail from Andalusia and can be served either hot or cold, before lunch or dinner, or as a meal or alone. Bars called *tascas* or *bodegas* specialize in *tapas* and offer patrons not only amazing appetizers, but also a fun way of socializing. *Spanish Gazpacho Soup Shooters* (First Courses, p. 57) and the *Spanish Potato Omelet* (p. 26) are examples of classic *tapas* offerings. Because Spanish menus are fairly traditional and tend not to change a great deal, creating new *tapas* offers Spanish chefs a fresh palette on which to create new culinary treats.

In Italy, fresh ingredients and simple, proven cooking styles are the keys to wonderful meals. There, appetizers are offered as a way to whet the palate and demonstrate the season's bounty of ingredients. Fresh vegetables and the catch of the day take center stage on Italian antipasto buffets and on restaurant menus. Many Italian *trattorie* (family-style restaurants) offer an appetizer plate, where diners can choose their appetizers the way Americans make salads at salad bars. *Bruschetta with Artichoke Purée and Roasted Red Peppers* (p. 27),

Eggplant Croquettes (p. 28), and *Marinated Italian Eggplants* (p. 29) are just a few of the traditional components of Italian antipasto bars.

In the eastern Mediterranean countries of Greece, Turkey, Lebanon, Syria, and Israel, many restaurants and taverns offer *meze* (appetizer) tables with both hot and cold dishes served on small plates. Their elaborate presentation and distinctive flavors are reminiscent of the imperial kitchens of the past. It is not uncommon for chefs to serve up to 40 different small dishes at a table or to make a buffet spread. *Carrots with Garlic and Yogurt* (p. 30), *Mixed Herb Plate* (p. 31), *Spicy Israeli Tomato Spread* (p. 33), *Fava Bean Purée* (p. 36), *Stuffed Vine Leaves* (p. 34), and *Fish Croquettes* (p. 37) are just a few of the many *meze* items available.

In the North African countries of Morocco, Tunisia, Algeria, Libya, and Egypt, appetizers are a symbol of hospitality and are used to heighten the appetite and build anticipation of the main course. There, appetizers usually consist of cold pulses, purées, salads, olives, and pickles, which are referred to by different names depending on the local diet. In Egypt, for example, all of the above items are collectively referred to as *salatat* (salads), even though most of them contain no lettuce. In Morocco, they are referred to as *kemia. Red Lentil Purée* (p. 39), *Roasted Eggplant Purée* (p. 40), *Traditional Chickpea and Tahini Purée* (p. 41), and *Tunisian Tuna, Tomato, and Egg Turnovers* (p. 44) are all examples of flavorful and healthful North African starters.

It is interesting and fun to offer various appetizers on small plates in place of a traditional meal. Try mixing and matching some of your favorites from various regions to come up with a menu that is your own. Keep in mind that small plates make wonderful buffet items and are perfect for entertaining.

This cool and refreshing purée makes a great alternative to fat-laden dressings on crudités platters. It can also be served warm with poultry and fish dishes.

Cool Carrot Purée with Bell Pepper Sticks

1. Cut carrots and celery into 2-inch chunks, and place in a heavy saucepan. Cover with water, and bring to a boil over high heat. Reduce heat. Simmer for 15 minutes or until fork-tender. Drain, place in a food processor, and pulse on and off. Add olive oil, lemon juice, and salt and pepper to taste. Purée until smooth. Refrigerate and serve cold or at room temperature with bell pepper sticks.

1 1/2 **lb carrots, peeled and trimmed**
   2 **celery stalks, trimmed**
   1 **Tbsp extra-virgin olive oil**
   2 **Tbsp lemon juice**
      Salt
      Freshly ground pepper
   2 **large green bell peppers, cut into thin slices**

Healthy Living Tradition

Carrots contain a great deal of vitamin A, which helps keep your skin and eyes healthy. To keep things easy, you can keep shredded carrots in a container in the refrigerator for up to a week. They can be added to salads and slaws. Diced carrots can be stored in plastic sandwich bags, making them ready to add whenever you need them.

Exchanges/Choices		Calories	15	Sodium	30mg
3 Vegetable		Calories from Fat	35	**Total Carbohydrate**	20g
1 Fat		**Total Fat**	4.0g	Dietary Fiber	6g
		Saturated Fat	0.6g	Sugars	10g
Serves 4		Trans Fat	0.0g	**Protein**	2g
Serving Size: 1/2 cup		**Cholesterol**	0mg		

Vegan dish

Although this simple dish is a popular appetizer in France, it also makes an excellent side dish. To serve as an appetizer, place purée in tiny ramekins and serve with crudités or crackers. To serve as a side dish, spoon into a bowl, and serve with *Poached Sea Bass with Tomatoes and Herbs* (p. 117), *Stuffed Chicken Breasts with Cucumber Cream* (p. 100), or *Veal Scaloppine with Roasted Red Peppers and Arugula* (p. 108).

Cauliflower and Broccoli Purée

1. Place cauliflower and broccoli in a large saucepan. Cover with water. Bring to boil over high heat, and cook 10–15 minutes or until tender. Drain well. Place vegetables in a food processor, and pulse on and off to form a rough purée. Stir in cheese. Taste, and season with salt and fresh pepper as desired.

2 cups cauliflower florets
4 cups broccoli florets
2 Tbsp Romano cheese
Salt
Freshly ground pepper

Healthy Living Tradition

Puréed cauliflower makes a tasty and nutritious alternative to butter-laden mashed potatoes. Keep frozen cauliflower on hand for an easy side dish.

Exchanges/Choices		Calories	30	Sodium	45mg
1 Vegetable		Calories from Fat	5	**Total Carbohydrate**	4g
		Total Fat	0.5g	Dietary Fiber	2g
Serves 6		Saturated Fat	0.3g	Sugars	2g
Serving Size: 1/2 cup serving		Trans Fat	0.0g	**Protein**	3g
		Cholesterol	0mg		

This is a very light French appetizer that can be served before a typical weeknight meal.

Celery Purée with Carrot Sticks

1. Place celery and carrots in a pot of water, and bring to boil over high heat. Reduce heat to medium. Cook for 30 minutes or until tender. Drain well, and place in a blender or food processor. Add lemon juice, salt, and pepper, and purée until smooth. Taste and adjust seasonings. Bring to room temperature, and refrigerate until cold. Serve with carrot sticks.

1	lb celery stalks, cut in half
1/2	lb carrot sticks, trimmed and cut in half
1	Tbsp lemon juice
1/2	tsp salt
1/4	tsp freshly grated pepper
	Carrot sticks, for serving

Healthy Living Tradition

After a long day, it's easy to be tempted to eat whatever is quick and handy when you get home. This recipe is great for curbing hunger while preparing a meal. I also like to keep Cool Carrot Purée with Bell Pepper Sticks (p. 20), Cauliflower and Broccoli Purée (p. 21), Red Lentil Purée (p. 39), Roasted Eggplant Purée (p. 40), Spanish Gazpacho Soup Shooters (p. 57), *and* Traditional Chickpea and Tahini Purée (p. 41) *in the refrigerator for the same reason.*

Exchanges/Choices		Calories	40	Sodium	415mg
2 Vegetable		Calories from Fat	0	**Total Carbohydrate**	9g
		Total Fat	0.0g	Dietary Fiber	3g
Serves 4		Saturated Fat	0.1g	Sugars	4g
Serving Size: 1/2 cup each		Trans Fat	0.0g	**Protein**	1g
		Cholesterol	0mg		
Vegan dish					

These savory pancakes are great appetizers and party dishes that the whole family will love. A dollop of olive paste, caviar, fish roe, tomato salsa, or sour cream makes a great garnish. If you take the salt and herbs out of this recipe and add 1 Tbsp sugar and fresh blueberries, you will have a delicious breakfast. This recipe can be made in large batches and frozen in resealable plastic bags. To serve, allow them to thaw, and reheat in a frying pan.

Cilantro Pancakes

1. Mix flour, baking powder, baking soda, and salt together in a large bowl. Add egg, yogurt, milk, and lime zest to dry mixture. Mix to combine, and stir in cilantro and dill. Whisk mixture with a wire whisk to incorporate all ingredients.

2. Heat olive oil in a large nonstick frying pan over medium-high heat. Pour batter into skillet in 4-inch round shapes. Allow pancakes to cook for 3–4 minutes or until bubbly and easy to turn. Flip pancakes over with a spatula, and cook for another 3–4 minutes or until lightly golden. Serve warm or at room temperature.

3/4	cup unbleached, all-purpose flour
1	tsp baking powder
1/4	tsp baking soda
1/8	tsp salt
1	egg
1/4	cup low-fat plain yogurt
1/4	cup nonfat milk
	Zest of 1 lime
1/2	cup fresh cilantro, finely chopped
1/4	cup fresh dill, finely chopped
5	tsp extra-virgin olive oil

Healthy Living Tradition

In North Africa, southern Europe, and the Middle East, fresh cilantro is used extensively for its distinctive herbal flavor. Fresh cilantro is actually easier to cook with than parsley because its stems are tender, and they don't need to be removed before adding them to recipes. Coriander (the dried seed from cilantro) is used to make tisanes.

Exchanges/Choices		Calories	170	Sodium	280mg
1 1/2 Starch		Calories from Fat	65	Total Carbohydrate	20g
1 Fat		**Total Fat**	7.0g	Dietary Fiber	1g
		Saturated Fat	1.3g	Sugars	2g
Serves 4		Trans Fat	0.0g	**Protein**	5g
Serving Size: 2 (4-inch) pancakes		**Cholesterol**	55mg		

This traditional Lebanese dish combines roasted eggplant with yogurt and pine nuts. It's silky, velvety texture and mellow taste make it an excellent alternative to mashed potatoes. When served with pita bread or crudités, this dish becomes a healthy and tasty appetizer.

Eggplant Caviar

1. Place a colander inside a bowl. Add yogurt. Set in the refrigerator for 6 hours or overnight.

2. Preheat broiler. Prick the eggplant in a few places with a knife, and place them on a baking sheet. Broil the eggplant for 20 minutes or until they are soft and wilted. Remove from the broiler, and let cool slightly.

3. When cool enough to handle, peel them with your fingers and slice off the tops. Place in a fine sieve or colander and press them gently to remove the juices.

4. Transfer to a medium bowl. Stir in drained yogurt and tahini. Taste, and season with salt and pepper, if necessary.

5. Heat olive oil in a small frying pan over medium heat. Add pine nuts, and toast quickly over low heat. Remove from heat when golden.

6. Spoon eggplant mixture onto a serving dish. Pour pine nuts and oil over the top. Serve warm or at room temperature.

1 cup whole-milk yogurt, drained overnight
2 lb eggplant
2 Tbsp tahini
1/2 tsp kosher salt
1/4 tsp freshly ground black pepper
1 Tbsp olive oil
2 Tbsp pine nuts

Healthy Living Tradition

This recipe calls for yogurt that has been drained overnight in a colander over a bowl. Draining yogurt produces a thick, spreadable, creamy cheese known as labna in Lebanon. This delicious concoction is so integral to Lebanese cuisine that the country's name is actually derived from it!

Exchanges/Choices	Calories	95	Sodium	130mg
1/2 Carbohydrate	Calories from Fat	55	**Total Carbohydrate**	9g
1 Fat	**Total Fat**	6.0g	Dietary Fiber	3g
	Saturated Fat	1.3g	Sugars	3g
Serves 8	Trans Fat	0.0g	**Protein**	3g
Serving Size: 1/4 cup	**Cholesterol**	5mg		

This quick, easy, and delicious appetizer never fails to impress guests. Molded "creamed" spinach can be served with *Spicy Israeli Tomato Spread* (p. 33) for a stunning red and green visual treat.

Spinach Flan

1. Preheat oven to 350°F.

2. Mix spinach, 1 Tbsp olive oil, lemon juice and zest, salt, pepper, and cheese together. Use remaining 1 Tbsp olive oil to oil the ramekins. Spoon spinach inside, and level off the tops. Bake for 20 minutes or until top of spinach begins to turn golden. Remove from oven. Using a pot holder, hold the ramekins in one hand and run a knife around the edges with the other to loosen. Hold ramekin perpendicular to a small plate, and unmold into the center. Serve warm.

3. If desired, spoon *Spicy Israeli Tomato Spread* around the sides of the spinach flan, and dollop a bit on the center of the top.

- 1 **(10-oz) package frozen spinach, thawed, drained, and chopped**
- 2 **Tbsp extra-virgin olive oil, divided**
  Juice of 1 lemon
  Zest of 1 lemon
- 1 **tsp salt**
- 1/4 **tsp freshly ground pepper**
- 2 **Tbsp Pecorino Romano cheese**
- 1 **recipe Spicy Israeli Tomato Spread (p. 33), if desired**

Healthy Living Tradition

Packed with nutrients, spinach is a great addition to any meal. To get more spinach in your daily diet, try the Calamari Stuffed with Spinach (p. 128)*;* Salmon Stuffed with Spinach and Feta (p. 122)*;* Bean, Lentil, and Spinach Skillet (p. 164)*;* Roasted Peppers Stuffed with Bulgur, Spinach, and Herbs (p. 70)*;* Romaine, Spinach, and Radicchio Salad (p. 172)*; and* Spinach-Stuffed Bread Triangles (p. 264)*.*

Exchanges/Choices	Calories	60	Sodium	445mg
1 Vegetable	Calories from Fat	45	Total Carbohydrate	3g
1 Fat	**Total Fat**	5.0g	Dietary Fiber	1g
	Saturated Fat	0.9g	Sugars	0g
Serves 6	Trans Fat	0.0g	**Protein**	2g
Serving Size: 1 ramekin	**Cholesterol**	0mg		

Tortilla de patatas **is one of Spain's most well-known culinary exports.** While small wedges of the omelet are traditionally served as an appetizer, they also make a great breakfast or accompaniment to soup and salad. **Try it with** *Red Lentil Soup* (p. 52) **and** *Orange, Asparagus, and Avocado Salad* (p. 168).

Spanish Potato Omelet

3 tsp extra-virgin olive oil
2 Russet potatoes (10 oz each), peeled and cut into thin slices
1/2 tsp kosher salt
3 eggs, lightly beaten

1. Heat the oil in a 9-inch nonstick frying pan over medium heat. Add the potatoes in a single layer (you will need to work in batches), and cook them slowly until they are tender on both sides (about 7 minutes per side). Remove from pan.

2. Continue with the next batch of potato slices. When all potatoes are cooked through, add reserved potatoes back to the pan. Season with salt. Add the eggs over the potatoes. Cover with a lid. When the edges of the omelet are cooked, place a large plate on top of the pan over the top and hold it with your hand. With the pan handle in your other hand, flip the omelet over onto the plate, and slide it back into the pan. Continue cooking for 5–10 minutes or until cooked through. Serve warm or at room temperature.

Healthy Living Tradition

When cooking and creating easy, healthy dishes, it's important to remember that you don't have to reinvent the meal wheel. Whenever you're ready for a change, simply add or substitute ingredients in recipes that you already enjoy. Onions, tuna fish, and peppers are popular additions to this omelet.

Exchanges/Choices	Calories	180	Sodium	300mg
1 1/2 Starch	Calories from Fat	65	**Total Carbohydrate**	22g
1 Med-Fat Meat	**Total Fat**	7.0g	Dietary Fiber	2g
	Saturated Fat	1.6g	Sugars	1g
Serves 4	Trans Fat	0.0g	**Protein**	7g
Serving Size: 1/4 omelet	**Cholesterol**	160mg		

This is my favorite way to serve bruschetta. The topping is an artichoke purée that I enjoyed while living in Rome, a city known for its love of artichokes. It is a typical antipasto served at one of my favorite pizzerias. Luckily, it's healthy and easy to make. Use the best-quality olive oil possible.

Bruschetta with Artichoke Purée and Roasted Red Peppers

1. With a large serrated knife, slice the bread into 6 (1.5 oz) slices on the diagonal. Lay the bread slices evenly on cookie sheets. Brush both sides with olive oil.

2. Place the artichokes, olive oil, lemon juice, cheese, salt, and freshly ground pepper into a food processor and process until a smooth purée is formed (less than 1 minute). Taste the purée, and adjust the seasoning, if necessary. Set aside.

3. Place the bread under the broiler. Toast for 3–5 minutes until golden. Turn bread over, and toast for another 3 minutes or until golden on the other side. Remove from the oven. Slather a thick layer of purée on each slice of bread. Top with red pepper slices. Serve warm.

1 **(10-oz) loaf crusty, day-old Italian bread**
1 **Tbsp extra-virgin olive oil**

Artichoke purée
1 **(14-oz) can artichoke hearts, drained and rinsed**
1 1/3 **Tbsp extra-virgin olive oil**
Juice of 1 lemon
2 **Tbsp Romano cheese**
Salt, to taste
Freshly ground pepper, to taste
1 **large roasted red pepper (from a jar), drained and thinly sliced**

Healthy Living Tradition

Keep this purée in a sealed container in your refrigerator for up to a week. Slather it on a slice of bread and eat it with an ounce of low-fat cheese for a quick and nutritious snack.

Exchanges/Choices		Calories	205	Sodium	475mg
1 1/2 Starch		Calories from Fat	65	Total Carbohydrate	28g
1 Vegetable		Total Fat	7.0g	Dietary Fiber	3g
1 1/2 Fat		Saturated Fat	1.4g	Sugars	3g
		Trans Fat	0.0g	Protein	6g
Serves: about 6		Cholesterol	0mg		
Serving Size: 1 slice (1.5 oz)					

Calabrian chefs and housewives are known for their ingenuity when it comes to creating delicious eggplant recipes. This recipe is one of my favorite appetizers. Serve it with tomato sauce for dipping.

Eggplant Croquettes

❋ Polpette di Melanzane ❋

1. Place bread in a small bowl, and cover with milk.

2. Place eggplant in a large saucepan, cover with water, and simmer for 20 minutes or until tender. Drain well. Place in a mixing bowl with 1 1/4 cup bread crumbs.

3. Squeeze milk out of bread, and add bread to the bowl with the eggplant and bread crumbs. Stir in cheese, parsley, basil, salt, and pepper. Mix well. Mixture should be thick enough to form balls; if it is too thin, add more bread crumbs until it holds together.

4. Pour remaining 1/2 cup bread crumbs into a shallow dish. Form teaspoons full of the eggplant mixture into 12 equally sized egg shapes. Roll eggplant into bread crumbs to coat.

5. Heat the olive oil in a large heavy skillet over medium heat. Add the croquettes to the skillet, leaving space between. Sauté for 3–4 minutes per side or until golden. Place eggplant balls on a platter, and serve hot with tomato sauce on the side for dipping.

2	slices (about 2 oz) day-old Italian bread, cubed
1/2	cup 1% milk
1	eggplant, chopped into 1/4-inch cubes
1 3/4	cup plain bread crumbs, divided
1/4	cup Pecorino Romano cheese, grated
3	Tbsp fresh Italian parsley, finely chopped
2	Tbsp fresh basil, finely chopped
1/8	tsp kosher salt
1/2	tsp freshly ground black pepper
1 1/2	Tbsp extra-virgin olive oil, divided
1	cup no-added-salt tomato sauce, for dipping

Healthy Living Tradition

This flavorful mixture can also be shaped into hamburger patties for an excellent alternative to traditional veggie burgers.

Exchanges/Choices		Calories	335	Sodium	580mg
3 Starch		Calories from Fat	90	Total Carbohydrate	52g
1 Vegetable		Total Fat	10.0g	Dietary Fiber	6g
1 1/2 Fat		Saturated Fat	2.3g	Sugars	9g
		Trans Fat	0.0g	Protein	11g
Serves 4		Cholesterol	5mg		
Serving Size: 3 croquettes					

The picture-perfect Sicilian town of Taormina is famous for its vegetable-based appetizers, natural springs, and serene spas. I've tweaked this recipe just a bit. Because eggplant skin contains antioxidants, potassium, magnesium, and fiber, I've chosen to leave it on in this recipe. In addition, I've replaced the traditional white wine vinegar with balsamic vinegar, which comes from northern Italy.

Marinated Italian Eggplants
❋ Melanzane Marinate ❋

1. Bring a pot of water to a boil over high heat. Add the vinegar. Add the eggplant, and boil for 5 minutes. Drain and rinse with cold water. Place the eggplant in a large bowl, and refrigerate for 1 hour or overnight.

2. To serve, toss eggplant with olive oil, garlic, mint, oregano, parsley, lemon juice, and salt and pepper to taste. Serve cold or at room temperature.

1/4 cup balsamic vinegar
4 baby eggplants (about 1 lb total), trimmed and diced into 1-inch pieces
3 Tbsp extra-virgin olive oil
4 cloves garlic, finely minced
2 Tbsp fresh mint, finely chopped
2 Tbsp fresh oregano, finely chopped
2 Tbsp fresh parsley, finely chopped
Juice of 1 lemon
Salt
Freshly ground pepper

Healthy Living Tradition

Fresh, in-season eggplant is a healthful and versatile vegetable. Choose shiny, smooth-skinned varieties that are free of bruises. The fresher the eggplants, the less bitter they will taste.

Exchanges/Choices	Calories	140	Sodium	5mg
2 Vegetable	Calories from Fat	90	Total Carbohydrate	12g
2 Fat	**Total Fat**	10.0g	Dietary Fiber	3g
	Saturated Fat	1.4g	Sugars	4g
Serves 4	Trans Fat	0.0g	**Protein**	1g
Serving Size: about 1/2 cup	**Cholesterol**	0mg		

Vegan dish

This delicious Turkish dish will make a carrot lover out of everyone. It has been adapted from Sheilah Kaufman's *A Taste of Turkish Cuisine.* It is traditionally served with olives.

Carrots with Garlic and Yogurt

❊ *Yoğurtlu Havuç* ❊

1. Place a colander inside a bowl. Add plain yogurt. Set in the refrigerator for 6 hours or overnight. Reserve juices (see Healthy Living Tradition).

2. In a large pot, heat 2 Tbsp olive oil over medium heat. Sauté the onions, stirring slowly, for 5 minutes. Do not let them brown. Add carrots, stirring to mix well, and cook for 10 minutes. Remove from heat, and let cool.

3. Crush the garlic and salt together in a mortar and pestle or with a knife on a chopping board.

4. Combine the cooled carrots with drained yogurt and garlic mixture in a large bowl.

5. In a small bowl, combine remaining 2 Tbsp olive oil and paprika. Pour mixture over the carrots, making a swirl design. Serve chilled or at room temperature.

2	cups plain yogurt, drained
4	Tbsp extra-virgin olive oil, divided
1	medium yellow onion, finely chopped
1	lb carrots, coarsely grated
4	cloves garlic
1/2	tsp salt
2	tsp paprika

Healthy Living Tradition

Don't discard the leftover liquid after draining the yogurt. In the eastern Mediterranean, refreshing drinks are made with this liquid and served on warm days.

Exchanges/Choices		Calories	110	Sodium	200mg
2 Vegetable		Calories from Fat	65	**Total Carbohydrate**	9g
1 1/2 Fat		**Total Fat**	7.0g	Dietary Fiber	2g
		Saturated Fat	0.9g	Sugars	5g
Serves 8		Trans Fat	0.0g	**Protein**	3g
Serving Size: about 1/2 cup		**Cholesterol**	0mg		

Arugula grows abundantly throughout the Mediterranean and Middle East. There, it is not seen as a gourmet food item, but as a staple, like lettuce or parsley. The leaves are served whole and sometimes garnished with a bit of the cooking sauce from fish. Otherwise, they are eaten without condiments.

Mixed Herb Plate

1. Immerse arugula in water in a large bowl. Drain and repeat until arugula is clean and no residue remains on the bottom of the bowl (this may take as many as seven washings). Dry arugula. Lay it on a large serving platter.

2. Trim ends off spring onions. Lay them on top of arugula. Arrange parsley or dill next to spring onions. Serve.

1 bunch fresh arugula
2 bunches spring onions
1 bunch fresh parsley or dill, washed and dried

Healthy Living Tradition

High in dietary fiber and containing a wide range of vitamins and minerals, spring onions are ideal for a healthy diet.

Exchanges/Choices		Calories	25	Sodium	20mg
1 Vegetable		Calories from Fat	0	**Total Carbohydrate**	5g
		Total Fat	0.0g	Dietary Fiber	2g
Serves 4		Saturated Fat	0.0g	Sugars	2g
Serving Size: 1/4 recipe		Trans Fat	0.0g	**Protein**	2g
		Cholesterol	0mg		
Vegan dish					

Yogurt is one of the traditional pleasures of Mediterranean kitchens. It's usually enjoyed for breakfast or as a light snack, with fresh figs and luscious mountain honey. The yogurt should be drained overnight for best results.

Cucumber, Yogurt, and Dill Salad

❋ Tzatziki ❋

1. Place yogurt in a medium colander over a bowl to drain overnight.

2. Place cucumbers in a colander and sprinkle with salt. Let stand for 20 minutes. Rinse off salt, and add cucumbers to yogurt. Stir in dill. Add garlic and onion, and season with salt to taste. Serve immediately to prevent salad from becoming runny.

- 3 cups plain low-fat organic yogurt, drained overnight
- 2 English cucumbers, peeled and diced
- 1/4 tsp salt
- 1/4 cup fresh dill, chopped
- 1 clove garlic, minced
- 1 small yellow onion, grated and drained

Healthy Living Tradition

After draining yogurt, you can enjoy the excess liquid as a refreshing drink.

Exchanges/Choices		Calories	60	Sodium	165mg
1/2 Fat-Free Milk		Calories from Fat	15	Total Carbohydrate	8g
1 Vegetable		**Total Fat**	1.5g	Dietary Fiber	1g
		Saturated Fat	0.7g	Sugars	4g
Serves 8		Trans Fat	0.0g	**Protein**	5g
Serving Size: 1/2 cup		**Cholesterol**	5mg		

This Middle Eastern classic is known by its Arabic name, *shakshouka.* **This recipe is adapted from Sheilah Kaufman's** *Sephardic Israeli Cuisine: A Mediterranean Mosaic.*

Spicy Israeli Tomato Spread

1. Heat the olive oil in a large skillet over medium heat. Add onion, and sauté until soft and translucent (3–5 minutes). Add the garlic, cook for a minute, and stir. Add tomatoes and peppers. Cover, and cook for 10 minutes. Add stock, tomato paste, salt, pepper, cumin, and chili pepper. Cover, and cook for 20–30 minutes, stirring occasionally.

2 Tbsp extra-virgin olive oil
2 medium yellow onions, diced
4 cloves garlic, chopped
4 tomatoes, coarsely chopped
2 large green peppers, chopped
1 cup low-sodium chicken or vegetable stock
3 oz tomato paste
Salt
Freshly ground pepper
1 tsp cumin
Pinch of chili pepper

Healthy Living Tradition

This spread is a healthful condiment that is a wonderful alternative to mayonnaise and other fat-laden spreads. Freeze it in ice cube trays, and cover well with plastic wrap. When needed, pop out one or two cubes, and thaw or heat them on the stove before serving.

Exchanges/Choices		Calories	80	Sodium	75mg
2 Vegetable		Calories from Fat	35	Total Carbohydrate	11g
1/2 Fat		Total Fat	4.0g	Dietary Fiber	3g
		Saturated Fat	0.5g	Sugars	5g
Serves 8		Trans Fat	0.0g	Protein	2g
Serving Size: 1/2 cup		Cholesterol	0mg		

Vegan dish

Plump stuffed vine leaves are usually served as side dishes and appetizers in North Africa and the eastern Mediterranean. Fresh vine leaves can sometimes be found at Middle Eastern and Greek grocers in spring. Otherwise, jarred vine leaves can be used. Stuffed vine leaves can be filled and rolled a day in advance and cooked the day of serving. They can also be made ahead of time, and stored for up to a week in the refrigerator. Because they can be served cold or at room temperature, they are perfect for entertaining.

Stuffed Vine Leaves

1. Place vine leaves in a large bowl. Cover with boiling water. Let stand for 10 minutes.

2. Finely chop the cilantro, parsley, and mint. In a medium bowl, mix rice, cilantro, parsley, mint, 3/4 cup tomatoes, onion, olive oil, salt, pepper, chili powder, and coriander.

3. Drain vine leaves. Place one leaf on a work surface, vein side up. Cut the excess piece of stem from the bottom of each leaf. Place 1 Tbsp filling in the middle of each leaf. Shape the filling to resemble the width of a pencil across the width of the leaf. Roll the leaf up, starting at the bottom. Tuck in the sides of the leaf as you go, making an envelope. Refrain from rolling the leaves too tightly or they will tear as the rice cooks and expands inside. Continue with remaining leaves.

1/2 lb fresh vine leaves or 1 (8-oz) jar preserved vine leaves, drained
1/3 cup fresh cilantro
1/3 cup fresh parsley
1/3 cup fresh mint
1 cup medium-grain rice, uncooked
1 cup canned or boxed, chopped or diced (no-sodium-added) tomatoes, divided
1 medium yellow onion (about 1/2 cup), grated
1/4 cup extra-virgin olive oil
1 tsp kosher salt
Freshly ground black pepper
1/4 tsp chili powder, if desired
1 tsp ground coriander
2 lemons, sliced

4. Place stuffed vine leaves, seam side down, next to each other in a heavy saucepan. They should be touching one another and fit into the pan without any spaces. Repeat a second layer on top, if necessary. Place a plate upside down on top in the saucepan to keep vine leaves from rising. Pour boiling water over the vine leaves until they are almost, but not completely, covered. Add the remaining 1/4 cup tomatoes and salt and pepper to taste. Cover and simmer on low heat until rice is fully cooked and leaves are tender (about 1 to 1 1/2 hours). To test the doneness, break one in half and taste it. Serve warm or at room temperature with lemon slices.

Healthy Living Tradition

This is one of the many recipes from the Mediterranean that is usually made communally. For entertainment and a new learning experience, invite friends and/or family to make this recipe with you.

Exchanges/Choices				
1 Starch	**Calories**	135	**Sodium**	175mg
1 Vegetable	Calories from Fat	45	**Total Carbohydrate**	21g
1 Fat	**Total Fat**	5.0g	Dietary Fiber	3g
	Saturated Fat	0.7g	Sugars	3g
	Trans Fat	0.0g	**Protein**	3g
Serves 12	**Cholesterol**	0mg		

Serving Size: about 3–4 vine leaves
(4 oz per serving)

Vegan dish

Fava beans are believed to be the world's oldest agricultural crop. One of the Pharaoh's favorites, this traditional Egyptian dish is still a popular breakfast and snack food. Egyptians regularly eat a breakfast of this dish, eggs, and pita bread to get all of the nutrients they need for an active day.

Fava Bean Purée

❋ *Fuul Medammes* ❋

1. Heat 1 tsp olive oil in a medium frying pan over medium-low heat. Add beans and juice from can, lemon juice, cumin, salt, and pepper. Stir well to combine. Cook for 5 minutes or until most of the liquid is absorbed. Reduce heat to low, and mash slightly with a fork or potato masher.

2. Spoon onto a serving plate. Make a hole in the center and drizzle remaining 1 tsp olive oil into it. Serve with a piece of pita bread. This dish can be eaten for a vegetarian lunch or dinner.

2 tsp extra-virgin olive oil, divided
1 (15-oz) can cooked fava beans (fuul medammes) with juice
1 lemon, juiced
1 tsp cumin
1/8 tsp salt
   Freshly ground pepper

TIP: Cooked fava beans may be purchased in the international aisle at most grocery stores or check the Where-to-Buy Guide for mail-order sources.

Healthy Living Tradition

Egyptians eat protein-packed breakfasts. This delicious dish is eaten for breakfast there. Look for high-protein, low-fat options to get your day off to a powerful start.

Exchanges/Choices		Calories	100	Sodium	555mg
1 Starch		Calories from Fat	20	**Total Carbohydrate**	14g
1 Lean Meat		**Total Fat**	2.5g	Dietary Fiber	4g
		Saturated Fat	0.4g	Sugars	6g
Serves 4		Trans Fat	0.0g	**Protein**	6g
Serving Size: 1/2 cup		**Cholesterol**	0mg		

Vegan dish

This recipe is my spin on flavorful *croquetas de pescado* (Spanish fish croquettes), which are served as an appetizer at tapas bars. They are simple to prepare and are a unique appetizer at parties.

Fish Croquettes

1. Combine fish, onion, parsley, Seafood Seasoning, and 1 Tbsp extra-virgin olive oil in a food processor. Purée until a smooth paste is formed.

2. Preheat oven to 375°F.

3. Place bread crumbs, almonds, paprika, and salt in a bowl, and stir to combine. Oil a cookie sheet with remaining 1 Tbsp olive oil. Transfer fish mixture to a bowl. Roll paste into 1-inch balls, and set on a platter. Roll in bread crumb mixture to coat. Place on baking sheet.

4. Bake for 30 minutes or until golden and cooked through. Serve hot, with lemon wedges.

- **3/4 lb boneless white fish fillets (cod, halibut, swai, halibut, tilapia, rockfish), cut into cubes**
- **1 yellow onion, quartered**
- **1/4 cup fresh parsley**
- **1 Tbsp Seafood Seasoning (p. 287)**
- **2 Tbsp extra-virgin olive oil, divided**
- **1/4 cup plain, dry bread crumbs**
- **1/4 cup blanched almonds, finely ground**
- **2 tsp sweet paprika**
- **3/4 tsp salt**
- **1 lemon, cut into wedges**

Healthy Living Tradition

Ground almonds are often added to breading mixes in Spain, which increases the nutrition level a great deal. Try replacing the bread crumbs in some of your favorite recipes with ground almonds.

Exchanges/Choices	Calories		185	Sodium	435mg
1/2 Carbohydrate	Calories from Fat		90	Total Carbohydrate	9g
2 Lean Meat	**Total Fat**		10.0g	Dietary Fiber	2g
1 1/2 Fat	Saturated Fat		1.2g	Sugars	2g
	Trans Fat		0.0g	**Protein**	15g
Serves 5	**Cholesterol**		30mg		
Serving Size: 3 croquettes					

The beautiful island of Corsica was ruled by Italy until the mid 19th century, when it became part of France. By combining both Italian and French country-style cooking with local specialties, Corsica developed a cuisine as awe inspiring as its scenery. Traditionally this recipe is made with fresh langoustines, which are shellfish that resemble miniature lobsters. In this recipe, colossal or jumbo shrimp can be used.

Corsican Prawns with Chickpea Cream

1. Place chickpeas, lemon juice, garlic, and 2 Tbsp olive oil in a food processor. Add 1/4 cup water, or enough to make a smooth purée.

2. Heat remaining 2 Tbsp oil in a large skillet over medium-high heat. Add prawns or shrimp, rosemary, chili flakes, salt, and pepper. Cook, uncovered, for 2 minutes per side or until prawns or shrimp turn pink.

3. Evenly spoon chickpea cream onto small plates. Flatten with the back of a spoon. Place prawns or shrimp on top, and serve immediately.

2 1/2 cups cooked or canned no-salt-added chickpeas, drained and rinsed
1/4 cup fresh lemon juice
2 cloves garlic, minced
4 Tbsp extra-virgin olive oil, divided
1 1/2 lb prawns or colossal or jumbo shrimp, peeled and deveined
2 tsp freshly chopped rosemary
Dash crushed red chili flakes
1/2 tsp kosher salt
1/4 tsp freshly ground black pepper

Healthy Living Tradition

I buy chickpeas in large quantities and use them to make delicious recipes all week long. I usually make one batch of this purée to serve one night, then add sesame paste to another batch to make hommus (p. 41), *which I can keep refrigerated, and keep plain cooked chickpeas in a plastic container in the refrigerator to add to salads, soups, and stews. This way, I get extra fiber and protein without a lot of work or planning.*

Exchanges/Choices			
1 Starch	**Calories**	195	**Sodium** 240mg
2 Lean Meat	Calories from Fat	80	**Total Carbohydrate** 15g
1 Fat	**Total Fat**	9.0g	Dietary Fiber 4g
	Saturated Fat	1.2g	Sugars 3g
	Trans Fat	0.0g	**Protein** 15g
Serves 8	**Cholesterol**	100mg	
Serving Size: about 1/3 cup purée			
+ 3 shrimp			

Lentils are a great source of protein, which is needed to build muscle. This dish offers a quick and flavorful way of serving lentils, because red lentils require less time to cook than other varieties.

Red Lentil Purée

1. Combine lentils, stock, tomato paste, garlic, salt, and freshly ground pepper in a medium saucepan. Bring to a boil over high heat. Stir, reduce heat to low, and cover. Simmer for about 20 minutes or until lentils are tender and all liquid is absorbed.

2. Transfer lentil mixture to a food processor and pulse on and off to form a paste. Return lentil purée to saucepan, and stir in coriander. Taste and adjust seasonings, if necessary. Place red lentil purée in a small bowl. Garnish with yogurt, and top with cilantro. If desired, served with toasted pita pieces. Arrange pita pieces on a plate and serve warm.

1 **cup dried red lentils, sorted and rinsed**
1 **cup fat-free, low-sodium vegetable or chicken stock**
1 **Tbsp tomato paste**
5 **cloves garlic, chopped**
1/2 **tsp salt**
   Freshly ground pepper, to taste
1 **Tbsp dried ground coriander**
1/4 **cup fat-free Greek yogurt, for garnish**
1 **Tbsp cilantro, for garnish**

Healthy Living Tradition

Add inexpensive, quick-cooking, nutritious red lentils to your favorite soup recipes for additional protein.

Exchanges/Choices				
1 1/2 Starch	**Calories**	175	**Sodium**	340mg
1 Lean Meat	Calories from Fat	5	**Total Carbohydrate**	30g
	Total Fat	0.5g	Dietary Fiber	11g
	Saturated Fat	0.1g	Sugars	3g
Serves 4	Trans Fat	0.0g	**Protein**	14g
Serving Size: 1/2 cup	**Cholesterol**	0mg		

Vegan dish

Called everything from "devil's eggs" to "apples of madness" in antiquity, the eggplant has gone from being one of the Mediterranean's most mistrusted to its most beloved vegetable. When purchasing eggplants, be sure to select ones that are shiny, bright, and free of bruises. Tahini is a paste extracted from sesame seeds. Because this dish is not heated, it's perfect for buffets and picnics. Using extra-virgin or unfiltered olive oil will improve the taste.

Roasted Eggplant Purée

❈ Baba Ghanouj ❈

1. Preheat broiler. Prick eggplants with a fork, and place on a baking sheet. Broil 15–20 minutes, turning once, until eggplants are blistered and collapse. Let cool. Peel and remove flesh. Place in a colander to drain. Press down with a fork until all liquid is removed. Place in a medium bowl.

2. With a fork, stir in tahini, salt, and lemon juice. (Tahini can be found in the international aisle in most supermarkets or near the peanut butter.) Gradually add olive oil until the texture resembles crunchy peanut butter. The amount of olive oil needed will depend on the water content and size of the eggplants used. (You should still see eggplant pieces in the purée. It should not be perfectly smooth.)

3. If desired, make a small well in the center and fill with olive oil (this additional oil is not included in the nutrition analysis). Garnish with parsley. Serve at room temperature with pita bread or crudités.

TIP: Roast eggplants a day ahead, and assemble this dish at the last minute.

- **2** eggplants (each 8–9 inches long)
- **2** Tbsp tahini
- **1/4** tsp salt
- Juice of 1 lemon
- **1 1/2** Tbsp extra-virgin olive oil
- **1** tsp freshly chopped parsley, for garnish

Healthy Living Tradition

Appetizers in the Mediterranean region are typically vegetable based. When entertaining, try using interesting and versatile ingredients like eggplants to start your meal.

Exchanges/Choices				
2 Vegetable	Calories	125	Sodium	160mg
2 Fat	Calories from Fat	80	**Total Carbohydrate**	11g
	Total Fat	9.0g	Dietary Fiber	3g
	Saturated Fat	1.3g	Sugars	3g
Serves 4	Trans Fat	0.0g	**Protein**	2g
Serving Size: 1/2 cup	**Cholesterol**	0mg		

Vegan dish

The word *hommus* means "chickpeas" in Arabic. The name for this dish, *hommus bil tahina*, translates to "chickpeas with sesame paste" in English.

Traditional Chickpea and Tahini Purée
❀ *Hommus bil Tahina* ❀

1. Place chickpeas in a food processor, reserving a few for garnish. Add the garlic, tahini, olive oil, salt, and cayenne pepper to the food processor. Purée until smooth.

2. Add water, tablespoon by tablespoon, until an extra creamy consistency is reached (you should need less than 1/4 cup in total). Scrape down the sides of the food processor, and purée for 1–2 minutes. Taste and adjust seasonings, if necessary.

3. If not serving immediately, store in a lidded container in the refrigerator. Otherwise, spoon into a small round dish. Using the back of a spoon, make dents in the top and fill the dents with olive oil (optional).

4. Sprinkle paprika, and arrange remaining chickpeas on the top. Serve with carrot sticks.

1 **cup cooked or no-salt-added canned chickpeas**
1 **clove garlic, minced**
1/3 **cup tahini (sesame purée)**
2 **tsp extra-virgin olive oil**
1/2 **tsp salt**
  Dash cayenne pepper, to taste
  Dash paprika, for garnish
  Carrot sticks, for serving

Healthy Living Tradition

Serve dips and purées with raw vegetable crudités instead of bread for a more nutritious snack or appetizer.

Exchanges/Choices	Calories	135	Sodium	210mg
1/2 Starch	Calories from Fat	80	Total Carbohydrate	10g
2 Fat	Total Fat	9.0g	Dietary Fiber	3g
	Saturated Fat	1.3g	Sugars	1g
Serves 6	Trans Fat	0.0g	Protein	5g
Serving size: 1/6 recipe	Cholesterol	0mg		

Vegan dish

These miniature calzones make a delicious, healthful snack or appetizer. The dough is made from a combination of whole-wheat pastry flour and all-purpose flour. In the Mediterranean, flour made from tender spring wheat berries is used for baking whole-wheat bread. In the U.S., that kind of flour is called whole-wheat pastry flour. Traditional whole-wheat flour produces tough dough and is not recommended for this recipe. Whole-wheat pastry flour can be found in most organic and specialty supermarkets. If you choose not to use this flour, use all-purpose flour instead. The filling for the calzones can be made a day ahead of time (see step 4) and stored in the refrigerator until ready to use.

Eggplant, Tomato, and Shallot Baby Calzones

❋ Calzone di melanzane e pomodori ❋

1. To make the dough, fill a liquid measuring cup with 2/3 cup warm water. Add the yeast and sugar, and stir. Let sit for 5 minutes, until bubbles appear. (If bubbles do not appear and the yeast does not look frothy, it is no longer fresh. Use new yeast.)

2. Place the flours and 1 tsp salt into a large bowl. Pour in the yeast mixture and 1 tsp olive oil. Mix well to form a smooth dough, and place it on a lightly floured work surface. Knead dough for 5–10 minutes or until it is smooth and elastic. (If dough sticks to your hands, add more flour a tablespoon at a time until it no longer sticks.)

3. Lightly dust a bowl with flour and place the dough in it. Cover with plastic wrap and a clean kitchen towel; let rise for 2 hours or until dough has doubled in volume.

1	tsp active dry yeast
	Pinch of sugar
1	cup whole-wheat pastry flour
1	cup unbleached all-purpose flour
1 3/4	tsp salt, divided
1/4	cup extra-virgin olive oil, divided
3	shallots (about 2 oz each), finely chopped
3	cloves garlic, finely chopped
1	medium eggplant (about 9 oz), cut into 1/2-inch cubes
1/2	cup diced low-sodium canned tomatoes
	Freshly ground pepper
3	oz part-skim shredded mozzarella

4. Meanwhile, or the day before, heat 1 Tbsp olive oil in a large, wide skillet over medium heat. Add shallots and garlic, stir, and cook for 2–3 minutes or until shallots are golden and tender. Stir in eggplant and tomatoes, and season with remaining 3/4 tsp salt and freshly ground pepper. Cook, uncovered, for about 10 minutes or until eggplant is tender. (This step can be done a day in advance.)

5. Line two baking sheets with parchment paper or silicone liners. Preheat oven to 425°F. When dough has risen, divide it in half. On a lightly floured surface, roll each piece out into a 10-inch circle. Using a pizza cutter, cut the dough into quarters, and shape each quarter into a circle. Place about 2 Tbsp filling in the middle of each circle. Lightly sprinkle some of the cheese on top. Fold the bottom half of the dough over the top. Press the edges of the dough over the filling to cover. Place on baking sheets. Repeat with remaining dough and filling.

6. Once all of the calzones are made and placed on baking sheets, brush the tops and sides with remaining olive oil. Using a knife, cut a small hole in the center of each so steam can escape. Bake for 20 minutes or until golden. Serve warm.

Healthy Living Tradition

The people in the Mediterranean region are able to get the most out of recipes by thinking of ways they can "extend" them into the future. This recipe has two easy time-saving uses so that in the time it takes to make this one recipe, you'll be making three. For example, the stuffing makes a wonderful side dish on its own. The dough quantity can also be doubled. After rising, it can be shaped into a ball and frozen. It can be defrosted overnight in the refrigerator, rolled out, and used to make a pizza whenever you need it. The finished calzones can also be frozen.

Exchanges/Choices		Calories	235	Sodium	580mg
2 Starch		Calories from Fat	80	**Total Carbohydrate**	32g
1 Vegetable		**Total Fat**	9.0g	Dietary Fiber	4g
1 1/2 Fat		Saturated Fat	2.1g	Sugars	2g
		Trans Fat	0.0g	**Protein**	7g
Serves 8		**Cholesterol**	5mg		
Serving Size: 1 (4-inch) calzone					

Home of picture perfect weather, beautiful beaches, and fantastic street food, the Tunisian island of Djerba is a popular vacation getaway for Europeans. One of Djerba's most celebrated street foods is *breik*, a deep-fried turnover filled with tuna and vegetables. This version is baked, making it easier and healthier for the home kitchen. I like to double the recipe and freeze half for another occasion. The turnovers make a great picnic item or appetizer and can transform simple soups and salads into tasty and interesting meals.

Tunisian Tuna, Tomato, and Egg Turnovers
❋ *Breik bil Toona, Tomatum wa Beid* ❋

1. Combine tomato, egg whites, tuna, onion, capers, salt, pepper, and parsley in a bowl. Mix well to combine. Preheat oven to 350°F.

2. Unfold phyllo sheets and stack on a work surface in a rectangle shape. Brush each layer lightly with olive oil. Stack three sheets on top of each other. Make five equally spaced vertical cuts down the length of the sheets. Place 1 tsp filling at the top of each strip. Fold the phyllo over the filling on the diagonal, leaving a straight edge on the bottom. Continue to fold the phyllo in a flag-folding fashion into a triangle (the way you would make a paper football). Continue with remaining phyllo and filling. Place finished turnovers on a baking sheet. Lightly brush the tops of the turnovers with olive oil.

3. Bake for 15–20 minutes or until golden. Serve hot, with lemon wedges.

- 1 Roma tomato, diced
- 3 large eggs, whites only
- 1 (6-oz) can tuna packed in water, drained
- 1 small yellow onion, grated
- 1 Tbsp capers, rinsed and drained
- 2 tsp salt
- 1/4 tsp freshly ground black pepper
- 1/4 cup fresh Italian parsley, chopped
- 9 sheets phyllo dough, thawed
- 1/4 cup extra-virgin olive oil
- 2 lemons, quartered

Healthy Living Tradition

Although many people associate phyllo dough with fattening desserts, it can also be used in savory applications like this one. The phyllo sheets themselves are harmless, and when brushed with olive oil instead of butter and baked instead of fried, they make a perfectly healthy indulgence.

Exchanges/Choices					
1/2 Starch	Calories	90	Sodium	425mg
1 Fat	Calories from Fat	35	Total Carbohydrate	10g
	Total Fat	4.0g	Dietary Fiber	0g
	Saturated Fat	0.5g	Sugars	1g
Serves 15	Trans Fat	0.0g	Protein	4g
Serving Size: 1 turnover	Cholesterol	5mg		

Favorite First Courses

Soups, Rice, Grains, Pasta, and Couscous

Soups

Throughout the Mediterranean, first courses are preferred in the form of smooth and creamy soups, rich and tender rice, puffy grains, plump pastas, and light, airy couscous. At one time, geography and economics dictated local customs, making first courses vary greatly from place to place. Nowadays, after millennia of trading with one another, Mediterranean cuisine has become a melting pot, and each of our five first course categories may be served anywhere.

Nevertheless, it is still important to understand the different cultural attitudes behind first courses. In France, North Africa, and the southern European and Middle-Eastern Mediterranean countries, soup is the most common way to start a meal. Rice, grain, pasta, and couscous dishes are accompanied by protein in the second course. Our modern American term for dinner, *supper*, comes from the French term *souper*, which means "to eat soup or dinner." Across the southern European portion of the Mediterranean, such as Portugal, Spain, France, and Italy, soups are generally served as part of light dinners accompanied by salad, bread, cheese, and olives. In these countries, people tend to eat the larger, multi-course meal at lunchtime, so *supper* is a light affair.

In North Africa, some southern European countries, and the Middle East, it is common to serve soups with the entrées at both lunch and dinner. More than one kind of soup may be served at the same meal. In these cultures, soup itself is not considered enough to constitute a complete dinner, no matter how rich or nutritionally balanced it is.

In our hurried modern lifestyles, I think there is room for implementing both traditions. Healthful simple soups should be a part of easy weeknight dinners. For weekends, holidays, and entertaining, however, more elaborate soups have the power to transform even the most basic meal into a celebration. This book contains succulent soup recipes that will add sizzle to your supper.

Rice and Grains

According to the U.S. Food and Drug Administration, "Diets rich in whole-grain foods and other plant foods and low in saturated fat and cholesterol may help reduce the risk of heart disease." The Mediterranean diet is full of whole grains and plant-food-based recipes that are low in saturated fat and cholesterol. Although grains themselves do not seem very glamorous, they are nutritional powerhouses that can help us look and feel our best. They are easy to find and inexpensive. Let this book guide you to expand your grain-cooking repertoire—your body will thank you!

Rice is the most commonly eaten grain in the entire world. It originally comes from Asia, where it was cultivated 6,000 years ago, and it still holds deep religious and cultural significance. Rice became popular in the Middle East after Alexander the Great introduced it. Egyptian rice and spices like saffron were imported to Spain by the Muslim Prince Abd al Rahman during the 9th century. Over the years, elaborate Arab recipes, such as *kabsah*, a saffron- and spice-infused meat and rice dish, were introduced. Rice and saffron soon became the star ingredients in *paella*, the ubiquitous Spanish rice skillet. The Spaniards then introduced the same variety of rice to Italy's Po Valley, where it was used to make *risotto*. When risotto was combined with saffron, it was transformed into the world-famous *risotto alla Milanese*. Nearby northern Italian cities usually serve different risotto recipes as a first course to their midday meals instead of pastas. Nowadays, almost each Mediterranean country has its own fragrant rice recipes, which are often substantial enough to be served alone.

In Greece and Turkey, rice is simmered with nuts, herbs, and spices as fragrant pilafs and vegetable stuffing. In the Middle Eastern and North African portions of the Mediterranean region, long-grain rice is mixed with beans, legumes, and spices, creating hearty vegetarian single-dish meals. Egyptians have their own unique short-grain rice, which is usually cooked with fried vermicelli for added color and taste. It is also used to stuff vegetables and is eaten daily.

Bulgur wheat is another popular product that usually comes from red winter wheat, which is boiled, dried, and cracked into pieces. It can be purchased in coarse, medium, and fine grades, which are often referred to as 3, 2, and 1, respectively, in Middle Eastern stores. Bulgur can be used in both sweet and savory applications, ranging from cereals and desserts to stuffing and salads. It is very popular in the Middle Eastern parts of the Mediterranean and is sold in the bulk section of most supermarkets and specialty stores.

Corn originally hails from Central America, where the Mayans, Aztecs, and Incas viewed it as sacred. Spanish explorers brought it back to the Mediterranean, where it was slowly and reluctantly incorporated into daily diets. Originally used as animal feed and prison food, corn-based products did not catch on immediately. In Latin America, corn was ground only after soaking it in lime or ashes overnight (a process that helps the body absorb niacin from the corn). Unfortunately, the Europeans who tried to eat corn as a primary part of the diet did not treat their corn before eating it, which resulted in widespread vitamin deficiencies, particularly in the American South. This created a mistrust of the crop, which continued into the early twentieth century. Today, it is a beloved ingredient in all cultures of the Mediterranean. In addition to eating corn in soups, stews, and salads, corn is used

to make cornmeal, or *polenta*, in northern Italy. Polenta is generally served as a base for a saucy main dish. It can also be transformed into sweet puddings and cakes. Today, corn oil is a close second to olive oil in popularity around the Mediterranean. Roasted corn is a popular street snack, and corn bread, cookies, and cakes are also enjoyed.

Pasta

In recent years, pasta has gotten a bad reputation as being an unhealthy food that people should avoid. What makes pasta problematic for Americans, however, is not the pasta itself. It is the enormous quantities in which it is served—which can greatly raise blood glucose levels—and the fact that it is laden with fattening meats and unhealthful store-bought sauces. The truth is, daily life in Italy is centered on the climax of the midday meal: a first course of simply and healthfully prepared pasta. Because pasta is generally served as a first course in a multi-course meal in Italy, it is served in small quantities. Sauces and condiments for the pastas vary daily. Local availability, the cook's whim, and tradition dictate how pasta is prepared.

On most days, however, various shapes of pasta are either served with light, airy, homemade vegetable and herb sauces or they are "dressed" with a combination of olive oil, garlic, herbs, and vegetables. Heavy meat, cheese, and cream-based sauces are typically reserved for holidays and special occasions. Italians typically do not eat pasta at dinner, because it is too heavy. By doing as the Italians do, eating small quantities of pasta with healthful toppings, you'll be able to include the pleasure of pasta in a diet perfect for anyone with diabetes.

Couscous

Couscous, Morocco's national dish, comes from the onomatopoeic Berber word *keskou*; it replicates the sound that the couscous makes while it is sifted.

In traditional communities, some women still gather to make couscous by hand. In Morocco, couscous truly is a staple food. It is often given to the poor and to local mosques as charity. Couscous is rarely served by itself, but rather as an accompaniment to meat, vegetable, poultry, or seafood stews.

When Sicily was under Muslim rule, couscous became a staple in the local diet as well. There, it is served with fresh seafood and a fragrant broth. Due to France's large North African population, couscous is now the number one food eaten outside of the home in France. Boxed varieties of instant couscous make it so easy to prepare that it is perfect for even the busiest weeknights. In addition to being used in savory applications, couscous makes wonderful sweet desserts as well.

This book contains 26 first-course recipes inspired by the cultures and cuisines of the Mediterranean. Created in the ubiquitous simple and straightforward Mediterranean style, these dishes are as much a delight to prepare as they are to eat. With tastes as tantalizing as these, you'll be able to cook up a luxurious culinary escape any time you wish. Fortunately, traditional Mediterranean-style recipes offer us the opportunity to eat for both pleasure and health.

Asparagus soup is a classic first course in Spain. Served in clear glasses or little mugs, it is a delicious and elegant starter. This soup is simple to make and reheats well.

Cream of Asparagus Soup

❋ *Crema de espárragos* ❋

1. Place asparagus, milk, and water in a large saucepan. Add salt and pepper. Stir. Bring to a boil over high heat. Cook, uncovered, for 8–10 minutes or until asparagus is tender.

2. Pour soup into a blender. Remove center spout from lid to prevent it from bursting. Place lid on blender, and hold a kitchen towel over the center hole. Purée until blended. Whip soup for 1 minute, and return it to the saucepan.

3. Heat soup over low heat until warm. Taste and adjust seasonings, if necessary. Pour into clear glasses or coffee mugs, and top with parsley.

2 bunches asparagus (about 1 lb), cleaned and trimmed
2 cups whole milk
2 cups water
1/4 tsp salt
Freshly ground pepper, to taste
4 Tbsp parsley, finely chopped

Healthy Living Tradition

Asparagus is bountiful during the spring and is used in a multitude of delicious dishes. It is packed with vitamins and minerals.

Exchanges/Choices				
1/2 Milk	Calories	100	Sodium	215mg
1 Vegetable	Calories from Fat	35	Total Carbohydrate	10g
	Total Fat	4.0g	Dietary Fiber	2g
	Saturated Fat	2.3g	Sugars	7g
Serves 4	Trans Fat	0.1g	Protein	7g
Serving Size: 1 cup	Cholesterol	10mg		

This soup is so smooth and silky. I like to serve it in clear glasses. The light green color is a perfect prelude to any spring meal.

Italian Asparagus Soup

✸ *Zuppa d'Asparagi* ✸

1. Place asparagus, milk, and water in a large saucepan. Add salt and pepper. Stir. Bring to a boil over high heat. Cook, uncovered, for 8–10 minutes or until asparagus is tender.

2. Pour soup into blender. Remove center spout from lid to prevent it from bursting. Place lid on blender, and hold a kitchen towel over the center hole. Purée soup until it is blended. Whip soup for 1 minute, and return it to the saucepan.

3. Add yogurt. Stir to mix well. Heat soup over low heat until warm. Stir in cheese. Taste and adjust seasonings, if necessary. Pour into clear glasses or coffee mugs, and top with parsley.

- 2 **bunches asparagus (about 1 lb each), cleaned and trimmed**
- 1 3/4 **cups nonfat milk**
- 2 **cups water**
- **Salt, to taste**
- **Freshly ground pepper, to taste**
- 1/4 **cup plain nonfat yogurt**
- 2 **Tbsp Parmesan cheese**
- 4 **Tbsp parsley, finely chopped**

Healthy Living Tradition

Asparagus is a leading supplier of folic acid, a crucial nutrient for developing healthy infants. A large spear has only 4 calories, so it can be enjoyed in abundance.

Exchanges/Choices	Calories	80	Sodium	105mg
1/2 Fat-Free Milk	Calories from Fat	10	**Total Carbohydrate**	11g
1 Vegetable	**Total Fat**	1.0g	Dietary Fiber	2g
	Saturated Fat	0.6g	Sugars	8g
Serves 4	Trans Fat	0.0g	**Protein**	8g
Serving Size: 1/4 recipe	**Cholesterol**	5mg		

During ancient times, Egyptians were the chief exporters of lentils in the world. Because lentils were traded for currency and their shape is reminiscent of small coins, they are often associated with wealth. Italians like to serve lentils on New Year's to wish their guests, and themselves, a prosperous, healthy New Year.

Tuscan Lentil Soup

❊ *Zuppa di Lenticchie* ❊

1. Heat olive oil in a large saucepan over medium heat. Add carrots, onion, and celery. Sauté until translucent (3–5 minutes), stir, and add lentils. Cook for 1 minute. Season with salt, if desired, and freshly ground pepper to taste. Add stock and parsley, stir, and increase the heat to high. When the stock begins to boil, reduce heat to medium low. Stir and cover. Simmer 45 minutes to 1 hour or until lentils are tender. Taste and adjust salt and pepper, if necessary. Garnish with basil. Serve warm.

1	tsp olive oil
2	carrots, diced
1	onion, diced
2	celery stalks, diced
1	cup brown lentils, rinsed
	Salt, optional
	Freshly ground black pepper
4	cups low-sodium vegetable or chicken stock
1/4	cup freshly chopped Italian parsley
1/4	cup fresh basil, finely chopped

Healthy Living Tradition

Make large batches of this soup, and freeze it in serving sizes. You'll have a nutritious alternative to canned soup whenever you need it.

Exchanges/Choices		Calories	210	Sodium	190mg
1 1/2 Starch		Calories from Fat	20	Total Carbohydrate	37g
1 Vegetable		Total Fat	2.0g	Dietary Fiber	13g
1 Lean Meat		Saturated Fat	0.3g	Sugars	7g
		Trans Fat	0.0g	Protein	13g
Serves 4		Cholesterol	0mg		
Serving Size: 1 cup					

Vegan dish

In addition to their attractive appearance, red lentils contain 13 grams of protein per 1/4-cup serving, cook quickly, and taste delicious. This is a simple yet elegant soup that is easy to serve on a busy weeknight, but has a refined taste worthy of guests.

Red Lentil Soup

1. In a large saucepan, heat oil over medium heat. Add onion, carrot, and celery. Sauté until vegetables are soft (5–10 minutes). Add lentils, stock, and salt. Stir and increase heat to high. Bring to a boil. Reduce heat to medium low, and simmer for 15–20 minutes or until vegetables and lentils are tender.

2. Carefully transfer soup to a blender. Cover with lid, and remove the center spout. Cover hole with a clean kitchen towel. Purée 1–2 minutes or until mixture is smooth.

3. Return soup to saucepan. Bring to a boil over high heat. Stir, reduce heat to low, and simmer, uncovered, for 10 minutes or until soup is slightly thickened. Serve hot.

1 Tbsp extra-virgin olive oil
1/2 cup diced yellow onion
1/2 cup diced carrot
1 medium celery stalk (about 1/2 cup), diced
1 cup red lentils, rinsed
6 cups low-sodium vegetable or chicken stock
1 tsp kosher salt

Healthy Living Tradition

For busy winter days, try packing this soup for lunch. It is a warm and healthy alternative to fast food.

Exchanges/Choices					
1 Starch	Calories	150	Sodium	475mg
1 Lean Meat	Calories from Fat	20	Total Carbohydrate	23g
1/2 Fat	Total Fat	2.5g	Dietary Fiber	8g
	Saturated Fat	0.4g	Sugars	4g
	Trans Fat	0.0g	Protein	8g
Serves 6	Cholesterol	0mg		
Serving Size: 1 cup				

Vegan dish

Harira is a traditional, hearty Moroccan soup that is eaten at sundown during Ramadan. *Harira* tends to thicken as it stands. If you are making this dish a day in advance, you may want to add more water or stock to it before reheating. This soup also freezes well.

Moroccan Harira Soup

1. Place onion in a large saucepan or stockpot. Add lentils, tomato purée, stock, saffron, coriander, salt, and pepper. Bring to a boil over high heat, stir, and reduce heat to low. Cover and simmer for 20 minutes.

2. Carefully remove the lid to avoid burning yourself with the steam. Add rice, celery, cilantro, parsley, chickpeas, and tomato paste. Stir, increase heat to high, and bring to a boil. Reduce heat to low. Cover and simmer for another 20 minutes or until vegetables and rice are tender and soup has thickened.

- 1 medium yellow onion, diced
- 1/2 cup lentils, sorted, rinsed, and drained
- 1/2 cup tomato purée
- 4 cups low-sodium vegetable stock or water
- 1/2 tsp saffron
- 1 tsp dried coriander
- 1/2 tsp salt
- 1/4 tsp black pepper
- 1/4 cup medium-grain rice
- 1 celery stalk, finely chopped
- 1/4 cup cilantro, roughly chopped
- 1/4 cup parsley, roughly chopped
- 1/2 cup chickpeas
- 1 Tbsp tomato paste

Healthy Living Tradition

Serve hearty soups like harira as main courses for dinner during the winter months. They're both satisfying and nutritious.

Exchanges/Choices		Calories	210	Sodium	455mg
2 Starch		Calories from Fat	10	Total Carbohydrate	40g
1 Vegetable		Total Fat	1.0g	Dietary Fiber	9g
1 Lean Meat		Saturated Fat	0.1g	Sugars	7g
		Trans Fat	0.0g	Protein	10g
Serves 4		Cholesterol	0mg		
Serving Size: 1 1/2					

Vegan dish

This creamy soup can be served as a first course or as part of a light supper with salad, bread, and cheeses. This recipe uses dried chickpeas, which need to be soaked overnight. If you don't have time to soak dried beans, you can substitute rinsed, no-salt-added canned beans. Doing this will also cut down the cooking time significantly.

North African Chickpea Soup
❋ Shurba bil Hommus ❋

1. Place chickpeas in a large saucepan or stockpot with 6 cups water and onion. Simmer, covered, on medium-low heat until chickpeas are tender (about 5 minutes for canned or 1 hour for dried chickpeas).

2. Remove from heat and drain, reserving cooking liquid. Place chickpeas in a blender. Add lemon juice, cumin, salt, and pepper. Blend well until a purée is formed.

3. Return mixture to pot. Taste, and adjust salt if necessary. If soup is too thick, stir in a few tablespoons of the cooking liquid. Stir and simmer on low heat until ready to serve.

1 **cup dried chickpeas, soaked overnight, rinsed, and drained well**
1 **medium yellow onion, thinly sliced**
1 **lemon, juiced (3–4 Tbsp)**
1 **tsp cumin**
  Salt, to taste
  Freshly ground black pepper, to taste

Healthy Living Tradition

Chickpeas are a good source of protein. Consider adding them to salads, soups, pastas, rice, and couscous dishes the way people in the Mediterranean region do to take advantage of the health benefits of chickpeas.

Exchanges/Choices			
1 Starch	Calories	125	Sodium 10mg
1 Lean Meat	Calories from Fat	20	Total Carbohydrate 22g
	Total Fat	2.0g	Dietary Fiber 6g
	Saturated Fat	0.2g	Sugars 5g
Serves 6	Trans Fat	0.0g	Protein 6g
Serving Size: 1 cup	Cholesterol	0mg	

Vegan dish

My favorite way of making tomato soup is to start with a traditional Italian tomato sauce as a base. The traditional Italian tomato sauce is the same as the one in the *Penne with Eggplant-Tomato Sauce* (p. 72). When making that recipe, you can make a double batch of the sauce, and reserve half of it before adding the eggplant to make this soup. In a pinch, you can use a good quality, low-sodium jarred tomato sauce to make the recipe.

White Bean and Tomato Soup

1. Heat oil in a large saucepan over medium heat. Add garlic. Sauté until it releases its aroma. Add tomato purée, salt, and pepper. Increase heat to high, and bring to a boil. Add parsley or basil. Stir, reduce heat to low, and cover. Simmer for 15 minutes. Remove lid carefully, and stir in stock and cannellini beans. Bring to a boil, uncovered, over high heat. Reduce heat to low, stir in orzo, and cook 10–15 minutes until pasta is *al dente*. Garnish with cheese, and serve hot.

- 1 **Tbsp extra-virgin olive oil**
- 3 **cloves garlic, minced**
- 1 **cup no-salt-added tomato purée**
  Kosher salt, to taste
  Freshly ground pepper, to taste
- 1/4 **cup freshly chopped parsley or basil**
- 3 **cups low-sodium vegetable or chicken stock**
- 1 **(15-oz) can low-sodium cannellini beans, drained and rinsed**
- 1/2 **cup orzo or other small pasta**
- 1/4 **cup grated Romano cheese**

Healthy Living Tradition

In Italy, the rinds of hard cheeses like Parmesan and Romano are added to soups and stews to add flavor. People buy blocks of cheese, grate it, and reserve the rinds for this purpose. If you have rinds at home, you can substitute them for the grated cheese in this recipe. If you prefer not to grate your own cheese, many specialty food stores now sell rinds alone. If you don't see them, ask the person at the cheese counter. A little bit of aged, flavorful cheese goes a long way!

Exchanges/Choices			
2 1/2 Starch	**Calories**	275	
1 Lean Meat	Calories from Fat	55	
1/2 Fat	**Total Fat**	6.0g	
	Saturated Fat	1.4g	
	Trans Fat	0.0g	
Serves 4	**Cholesterol**	5mg	
Serving Size: 1 cup			

Sodium	180mg
Total Carbohydrate	43g
Dietary Fiber	7g
Sugars	6g
Protein	12g

Fresh tomatoes and herbs are as important to summer Mediterranean menus as they are to American ones. This light, piquant French soup is a wonderful predecessor to grilled or roasted chicken. It also tastes great with sandwiches and can be served chilled. Try packing it in a thermal carafe and serving it in cups at a picnic.

Chilled Tarragon and Tomato Soup
❊ *Soupe de Tomates et Estragon* ❊

1. Place the entire contents of tomato cans, balsamic vinegar, sugar, lemon juice, and 3 Tbsp tarragon in a food processor or blender. Mix to form a smooth sauce.

2. Place a large, fine-mesh strainer over a bowl. Use a wooden spoon to turn and press the sauce through a little at a time, until the tomato solids are left in the strainer and the juice has passed through (see Healthy Living Tradition).

3. Place the sauce in a large saucepan. Season with pepper to taste. Bring mixture to a boil over high heat. Reduce heat to low. Simmer, uncovered, for 10–20 minutes or until soup has thickened and has been reduced by about one-third of its original volume. Garnish with remaining tarragon leaves. Serve warm.

3 (14.5-oz) cans fire-roasted diced tomatoes
2 tsp balsamic vinegar
1 tsp sugar
1 tsp lemon juice
4 Tbsp finely chopped tarragon leaves, divided
Freshly ground pepper

Healthy Living Tradition

Part of the joy of Mediterranean cooking is challenging yourself to come up with the best use of leftover ingredients. Reserve the tomato solids from the strainer. Use them to mix with plain yogurt for a tasty vegetable dip, or spread them on thinly sliced baguettes to make bruschetta. They also make a great topping for sandwiches and can be added to stews. See how many delicious ideas you can come up with from leftover ingredients and apply this technique to other recipes.

Exchanges/Choices		Calories	70	Sodium	640mg
3 Vegetable		Calories from Fat	5	Total Carbohydrate	13g
		Total Fat	0.5g	Dietary Fiber	1g
		Saturated Fat	0.1g	Sugars	9g
Serves 4		Trans Fat	0.0g	Protein	2g
Serving Size: 3/4–1 cup		Cholesterol	0mg		
Vegan dish					

Gazpacho is the traditional soup of Andalucía, a region in Southern Spain known for its vibrant, sun-drenched cuisine. This soup is ideal for summer, because it requires no cooking. Try serving it as an appetizer at your next barbecue or picnic—soup in glasses is always fun. For this recipe, use clear glasses that hold 1/2 cup of liquid for appetizers or larger glasses or bowls for lunch or dinner first courses. Keep in mind that this soup needs to be refrigerated a minimum of 8 hours or overnight to allow flavors to develop.

Spanish Gazpacho Soup Shooters

1. Place all ingredients in a food processor or blender. (If necessary, add in batches). Purée until smooth. If needed, add water a tablespoon at a time until desired thickness is reached. Soup should be slightly thick, yet drinkable. Refrigerate at least 8 hours or overnight before serving.

3 cups no-sodium-added boxed chopped tomatoes
1 cup cubed Italian or French bread
1 medium cucumber, peeled and diced
1 small yellow onion (about 1/4 cup), chopped
1 green bell pepper, seeded and chopped
2 cloves garlic, chopped
2 Tbsp extra-virgin olive oil
1/2 cup low-sodium vegetable or chicken stock
2 Tbsp distilled white vinegar
3/4 tsp kosher salt
1/2 tsp black pepper

Healthy Living Tradition

This dish can also work as a flavorful and fun appetizer. By serving just a 1/2 cup per person, you can whet the appetites of 10 people!

Exchanges/Choices					
1/2 Starch	Calories	125	Sodium	430mg
2 Vegetable	Calories from Fat	55	**Total Carbohydrate**	17g
1 Fat	**Total Fat**	6.0g	Dietary Fiber	4g
	Saturated Fat	0.8g	Sugars	7g
	Trans Fat	0.0g	**Protein**	3g
Serves 5	**Cholesterol**	0mg		
Serving Size: 1 cup				

Vegan dish

Almonds are one of nature's gifts to the Mediterranean. They are eaten fresh and used in milk, soups, garnishes, and delicious desserts. This popular Spanish soup is made from ground almonds and bread. It is often called "white gazpacho." It's healthy, easy to make, and refreshing. Just remember that it needs to chill for a few hours before serving.

White Gazpacho Mocktails

1. Place bread in a bowl. Pour 1/2 cup water over it. Let stand 5 minutes. Place bread in a strainer. Squeeze out excess water, and transfer to a food processor. Add almonds, garlic, olive oil, lemon juice, vinegar, salt, and pepper. Pulse on and off to combine ingredients. Slowly add in 2 cups water, and continue processing until mixture is smooth. Transfer to a bowl, cover, and refrigerate overnight or for at least 6 hours. Serve 1/2 cup soup in martini or cocktail glasses with halved grapes on top.

- **4 oz day-old Italian or French bread, cubed**
- **1 cup blanched almonds**
- **2 cloves garlic, minced**
- **1 Tbsp extra-virgin olive oil**
- **3 Tbsp lemon juice**
- **1 tsp vinegar**
- **1/4 tsp salt**
- **1/4 tsp freshly ground pepper**
- **12 seedless green or black grapes, for garnish**

Healthy Living Tradition

The "good fat" in almonds can help promote heart health, and this makes them an excellent addition to the diet. Be sure to choose raw, unsalted ones.

Exchanges/Choices				
1 Carbohydrate	**Calories**	220	**Sodium**	220mg
1 Lean Meat	Calories from Fat	135	**Total Carbohydrate**	17g
2 1/2 Fat	**Total Fat**	15.0g	Dietary Fiber	3g
	Saturated Fat	1.4g	Sugars	4g
	Trans Fat	0.0g	**Protein**	7g
Serves 6	**Cholesterol**	0mg		
Serving Size: 1/2 cup				

Most North African and Middle Eastern countries have a favorite spiced chickpea dish. In addition to its taste, cumin is added to cooking legumes in order to make them easier to digest and rid them of their gas-producing qualities. Preserved lemons can be found in Mediterranean and Middle Eastern markets, as well as the international aisle of most specialty supermarkets. If you do not have them, substitute fresh-squeezed lemon juice. Serve with *Saffron Couscous* (p. 76) and *Carrot, Date, and Orange Salad* (p. 176) for a quick, easy, and delicious North African meal.

Spicy Tunisian Chickpea Stew

❋ *Tajine Hommus* ❋

1. If using dried chickpeas, place in a pot and cover with water. Bring to a boil over high heat, and reduce heat to low. Simmer for 1 1/2–2 hours or until tender. (This step can be done up to a week in advance).

2. Place chickpeas in a bowl of cold water. Rub them with your hands to remove skins.

3. Heat olive oil in a large skillet over medium heat. Add the onion and garlic. Sauté over low heat for 10 minutes or until golden. Add chickpeas, tomatoes, cumin, coriander, paprika, and crushed red pepper. Add stock, stir, increase heat to high, and bring to a boil. Reduce heat to medium low. Simmer for 40 minutes or until chickpeas are tender. Add preserved lemons, increase heat to high, and cook for 5 minutes, uncovered, or until most of liquid is absorbed. To serve, sprinkle with parsley.

1 cup dried chickpeas, soaked overnight, or 2 (14-oz) cans reduced-sodium chickpeas
2 Tbsp extra-virgin olive oil
1 large yellow onion, diced
1 clove garlic, minced
1/2 cup no-salt-added diced tomatoes
1 tsp ground cumin
1 tsp ground coriander
1 tsp paprika
Pinch dried crushed red pepper
1 1/2 cups fat-free, low-sodium vegetable stock
2 preserved lemons, quartered
2 Tbsp freshly chopped parsley

Healthy Living Tradition

Because dried chickpeas contain less sodium, they are more healthful than canned varieties. Of course, they take longer to prepare. I like to cook large batches at a time, and store them in serving-size quantities in the refrigerator. Whenever I need them, they're ready for me. Dried chickpeas are also less expensive.

Exchanges/Choices			
2 Starch • 1 Vegetable	Calories	275	Sodium	80mg
1 Lean Meat • 1 Fat	Calories from Fat	90	Total Carbohydrate	38g
	Total Fat	10.0g	Dietary Fiber	10g
Serves 4 / Serving Size: 1/2 cup	Saturated Fat	1.2g	Sugars	9g
	Trans Fat	0.0g	Protein	10g
Vegan dish	Cholesterol	0mg		

The ancient Egyptians used garlic as an antibiotic, to heal wounds, to ward off illness and evil spirits, and as a culinary ingredient. Today, chefs continue to be inspired by garlic's multitude of virtues. This Spanish soup makes a light first course in a meal of substantial dishes like the *Spanish Potato Omelet* (p. 26) and *Valencian Seafood Paella* (p. 130).

Spanish Garlic Soup

❋ *Sopas de Ajo* ❋

1. Heat oil in a large pot over medium heat. Add garlic. When garlic begins to turn color, add bread. Stir with a wooden spoon. Add paprika, water, and salt to taste. Increase heat to high. Bring to a boil, reduce heat to low, and simmer, covered, for 10 minutes. Serve hot.

2 **Tbsp extra-virgin olive oil**
6 **cloves garlic, peeled and minced**
2 **pieces (about 7 oz total) day-old country bread, cut into cubes**
1 **tsp sweet paprika**
4 **cups boiling water**
  Salt, to taste

Healthy Living Tradition

Broth-based soups are friends to gourmands and the diet conscious alike. Use them as a first course for nutritional value and to fill up more quickly.

Exchanges/Choices	Calories	205	Sodium	300mg
2 Starch	Calories from Fat	80	**Total Carbohydrate**	27g
1 Fat	**Total Fat**	9.0g	Dietary Fiber	2g
	Saturated Fat	1.3g	Sugars	1g
Serves 4	Trans Fat	0.0g	**Protein**	5g
Serving Size: 3/4 cup	**Cholesterol**	0mg		

In Italy, a *minestra* is a thick soup made from a multitude of ingredients. Adding the suffix *-one* on the end means that it is a "large or big" *minestra*, which explains why there are so many ingredients in this recipe. To make this dish vegetarian, substitute vegetable stock for the chicken stock.

Traditional Minestrone

1. Heat olive oil in a large stockpot over medium heat. Add onion, carrots, and celery, and stir. Sauté for 3–5 minutes or until tender. Add parsley and garlic. Cook for 1 minute longer. Stir in cabbage and potatoes. Pour in chicken stock, increase heat to high, and bring to a boil. Add zucchini, tomatoes, string beans, and cannellini beans. Stir in vinegar. Cover and allow to simmer for 40 minutes to 1 hour or until vegetables are tender. Taste, and add salt and pepper, if necessary.

2. Use a ladle to transfer half of the soup to a blender. Remove the spout on the lid, and cover with a folded kitchen towel. Purée until smooth, and return to stockpot. Stir to blend. Serve hot, topped with cheese.

1 Tbsp extra-virgin olive oil
1 medium yellow onion, finely chopped
2 carrots, finely chopped
1 celery stalk, finely chopped
1/4 cup flat-leaf parsley, chopped
6 cloves garlic, chopped
3 cups shredded cabbage
1 Yukon gold potato, peeled and chopped into bite-size pieces
8 cups low-sodium chicken stock
2 zucchini, peeled and chopped into bite-size pieces
2 large tomatoes, chopped
1/2 lb string beans, chopped into bite-size pieces
1 (15-oz) can no-salt-added cannellini beans
2 Tbsp balsamic vinegar
Salt, to taste
Freshly ground pepper, to taste
1/2 cup freshly grated Parmesan cheese

Healthy Living Tradition

Hearty yet low-calorie soups like this one are perfect for filling up without using fattening ingredients.

Exchanges/Choices			
1/2 Starch	Calories	130	
2 Vegetable	Calories from Fat	30	
1/2 Fat	**Total Fat**	3.5g	
	Saturated Fat	1.1g	
	Trans Fat	0.0g	
Serves 10	**Cholesterol**	5mg	
Serving Size: about 1 cup			

Sodium	475mg
Total Carbohydrate	19g
Dietary Fiber	5g
Sugars	5g
Protein	8g

This simple yet elegant soup is perfect with salad, bread, and cheeses for a light dinner.

Potato and Herb Soup

1. Heat olive oil over medium heat in a large saucepan or stockpot. Add potatoes and brown on all sides. Stir in parsley, stock, salt, and pepper. Increase heat to high, and bring to a boil. Reduce heat to low, cover, and simmer 20–30 minutes or until potatoes are tender.

1 **Tbsp extra-virgin olive oil**
4 **Russet potatoes, cubed**
1 **cup finely chopped fresh parsley**
8 **cups low-sodium vegetable or chicken stock**
   Salt, to taste
   Freshly ground pepper, to taste

Healthy Living Tradition

Easy soups like this one can be made in large batches and frozen in individual serving sizes. They are a healthy and fresh alternative to canned soups.

Exchanges/Choices		Calories	145	Sodium	200mg
2 Starch		Calories from Fat	20	**Total Carbohydrate**	28g
		Total Fat	2.5g	Dietary Fiber	4g
Serves 6		Saturated Fat	0.3g	Sugars	3g
Serving Size: 1 1/2 cups		Trans Fat	0.0g	**Protein**	3g
		Cholesterol	0mg		
Vegan dish					

This simple recipe transforms humble pantry ingredients into a soothing, buttery soup.

Yogurt and Potato Soup

1. Place a colander inside a bowl. Add yogurt. Set in the refrigerator for 6 hours or overnight.

2. Pour vegetable stock into a large stockpot. Bring to a boil over high heat. Add salt to taste and potatoes. Reduce heat to low, and simmer for 5–10 minutes or until potatoes are tender. Turn off the heat.

3. In a small saucepan, whisk together the drained yogurt, milk, and egg over medium heat. Bring the mixture to a boil, vigorously whisking the entire time. In a small bowl, combine the olive oil and paprika. When the yogurt mixture boils, stir in the oil-paprika mixture.

4. Place potato soup over medium heat. Slowly whisk in the yogurt mixture. Simmer for 5 minutes, and serve hot.

- 5 Tbsp plain, fat-free yogurt, drained overnight
- 4 cups fat-free, low-sodium vegetable stock
  Kosher salt, to taste
- 1 lb (about 3 medium) Yukon Gold potatoes, diced
- 1/2 cup nonfat milk
- 1 large egg
- 1 Tbsp extra-virgin olive oil
- 1/2 tsp paprika

Healthy Living Tradition

Yogurt can be substituted for heavy cream and sour cream in many recipes. It adds creaminess without the fat.

Exchanges/Choices	Calories	195	Sodium	190mg
2 Starch	Calories from Fat	45	**Total Carbohydrate**	31g
1 Fat	**Total Fat**	5.0g	Dietary Fiber	3g
	Saturated Fat	0.9g	Sugars	5g
Serves 4	Trans Fat	0.0g	**Protein**	6g
Serving Size: about 1 cup	**Cholesterol**	55mg		

Escarole is a broad-leaf endive related to the chicory family. Popular in Italian cuisine, escarole can be eaten raw like lettuce, sautéed, or added to soups and stews. It contains significant amounts of vitamins A and C and is higher in nutrients than radicchio. This is an everyday version of Italian wedding soup—the kind of satisfying soup that is a great meal on its own. For an extra treat, serve this soup with *Rosemary Focaccia* (p. 260) or *Rustic Dinner Rolls* (p. 256).

Escarole and Meatball Soup

1. Grease a baking sheet with olive oil. Preheat the oven to 350°F. Pour 1/4 cup water onto the bottom of the baking sheet. Set aside.

2. Mix bread crumbs, chicken, onion, garlic, cilantro, coriander, 1/4 tsp salt, a few twists of freshly ground pepper, and mustard in a medium bowl. Roll the mixture into 1-inch balls. Place on the baking sheet.

3. Bake meatballs in the center of the oven for about 30 minutes or until cooked through.

4. Bring stock to a boil in a large pan. Reduce heat to medium. Add meatballs, escarole, chickpeas, and red pepper flakes. Cook for 5–10 minutes or until escarole is wilted and tender.

- **1 tsp extra-virgin olive oil**
- **1/2 cup plain, dry bread crumbs**
- **1 lb ground chicken**
- **1 medium yellow onion, finely chopped**
- **3 cloves garlic, minced**
- **1 bunch fresh cilantro, finely chopped**
- **1 tsp ground coriander**
- **1/4 tsp salt**
  Freshly ground pepper, to taste
- **1 tsp Dijon mustard**
- **6 cups low-sodium chicken stock**
- **1 head escarole (about 3/4 lb), cut into 1-inch pieces**
- **1 (15-oz) can low-sodium chickpeas, rinsed and drained**
- **1/4 tsp dried crushed red pepper flakes**

Healthy Living Tradition

Cilantro adds an unexpected burst of flavor. This flavor is further deepened by adding its seeds, coriander. Don't worry about trimming cilantro in recipes, the stems are tender and can be eaten. Try substituting it for parsley in your favorite recipes and serving it chopped in raw salads.

Exchanges/Choices				
1 Starch • 1 Vegetable	**Calories**	260	**Sodium**	335mg
3 Lean Meat • 1/2 Fat	Calories from Fat	80	**Total Carbohydrate**	25g
	Total Fat	9.0g	Dietary Fiber	6g
	Saturated Fat	2.2g	Sugars	4g
Serves 6	Trans Fat	0.0g	**Protein**	22g
Serving Size: about 1 1/2 cups soup	**Cholesterol**	60mg		
+ 6 meatballs				

Sicily is known for its large, substantial salads, which were portable meals for farmers, shepherds, and fishermen. This is a tasty salad that can be made a day ahead of time. The rice and peas must be cooked until they are *al dente*, cooked through but still firm, or else the salad will be mushy.

Arborio Rice Salad with Vegetables

1. Bring water to a boil over high heat in a medium saucepan. Add 1/4 tsp salt. Add rice, lower heat to medium, and cook for 10–15 minutes, until tender, yet still firm to the bite (*al dente*).

2. Bring another medium saucepan of water to a boil over high heat. Add 1/4 tsp salt. Add peas. Boil for 3–5 minutes or until cooked, but not mushy.

3. Drain rice and peas. Rinse with cold water. Transfer to a bowl, and stir in 1 Tbsp olive oil.

4. Heat remaining oil in a large skillet over medium heat. Add onion, and sauté until golden. Add beans, vinegar, lemon juice, mustard, tomatoes, lemon zest, capers, mint, olives, and cucumbers. Cook for 1 minute. Remove from heat. Allow to cool to room temperature.

5. Stir bean mixture into rice and pea mixture. Serve at room temperature or refrigerate for up to 1 day and serve cold.

- 1/2 tsp sea or kosher salt, divided
- 3/4 cup Arborio rice
- 1 cup fresh English peas
- 3 Tbsp extra-virgin olive oil, divided
- 1 small yellow onion, finely chopped
- 1 (15-oz) can no-salt-added cannellini beans, drained and rinsed
- 1 Tbsp distilled white vinegar
- 1/3 cup freshly squeezed lemon juice (about 2 lemons)
- 1 tsp Dijon mustard
- 1/3 cup boxed chopped tomatoes or diced cherry tomatoes
  Zest of 2 lemons
- 1 tsp capers, rinsed and drained
- 1/2 cup fresh mint, finely chopped
- 1/4 cup black olives, pitted and cut into quarters
- 1 English cucumber, diced

Healthy Living Tradition

To maximize the benefits of vegetarian dishes, learn how to combine them properly to make complete proteins. By combining rice or other grains with peas, legumes, or beans, you can get all of the essential amino acids present in a complete protein without having to eat meat.

Exchanges/Choices			
1 1/2 Starch	Calories	165	Sodium 105mg
1 Vegetable	Calories from Fat	45	Total Carbohydrate 25g
1/2 Fat	Total Fat	5.0g	Dietary Fiber 4g
	Saturated Fat	0.8g	Sugars 4g
	Trans Fat	0.0g	Protein 5g
Serves 9	Cholesterol	0mg	
Serving Size: 1/2 cup			

Vegan dish

This fluffy, fragrant dish is a perfect alternative to plain or fried rice. High-quality saffron will give the rice a beautiful yellow color, and the cinnamon will give the dish a greater depth of flavor. In India, basmati rice is known as the "prince of rice" because of its delicious taste and high quality.

Saffron Rice with Almonds and Raisins

1. Combine rice, chicken stock, saffron, and cinnamon in a large saucepan over high heat. Bring to a boil. Reduce heat to low, and cover with a tight-fitting lid that has been wrapped tightly in a clean kitchen towel to absorb excess moisture. Simmer until all liquid is absorbed and rice is fluffy (15–20 minutes).

2. While the rice is cooking, warm a small skillet over medium heat. Add almonds and raisins to the skillet. Sauté for 2–4 minutes, until the nuts release their aroma and raisins are plump. Stir and make sure that all of the almonds are toasted. Remove from heat, and set aside.

3. When rice has finished cooking, let it stand, covered, for 10 minutes. Fluff it with a fork, remove cinnamon stick, and spoon into a serving bowl. Garnish with toasted almonds and raisins. Serve hot.

- 2 **cups basmati rice, soaked for 20 minutes and drained**
- 3 1/2 **cups low-sodium chicken or vegetable stock**
- 1/2 **tsp saffron, crushed**
- 1 **cinnamon stick**
- 2 **Tbsp slivered almonds**
- 2 **Tbsp raisins**

Healthy Living Tradition

Rice and couscous dishes are greatly enhanced by a simple sprinkling of toasted nuts and raisins. Try toasting a cup of each at a time, combining them, and tossing a few tablespoons on top of your next dish as a garnish. They will last up to a month in a sealed container in the refrigerator.

Exchanges/Choices		Calories	185	Sodium	40mg
2 1/2 Starch		Calories from Fat	15	**Total Carbohydrate**	37g
		Total Fat	1.5g	Dietary Fiber	1g
Serves 8		Saturated Fat	0.3g	Sugars	2g
Serving Size: 1/2 cup		Trans Fat	0.0g	**Protein**	5g
		Cholesterol	0mg		
Vegan dish					

This dish was probably introduced to the Middle East when basmati rice was imported from India. Basmati rice quickly gained popularity because of its fragrant flavor and fluffy texture. Serve this dish with the *Cucumber, Yogurt, and Dill Salad* (p. 32).

Chickpeas and Rice

1. If using dried chickpeas, place in a pot and cover with water. Bring to a boil over high heat, and reduce heat to low. Simmer for 1 1/2–2 hours or until tender. (This step can be done up to a week in advance).

2. In a medium saucepan, combine chickpeas, stock or water, salt, and pepper. Cook, uncovered, for 15 minutes over medium heat. Add rice and cumin. Mix well. Reduce heat to low, and cover. Cook until rice is tender and liquid is absorbed, 20–30 minutes.

3. While rice is cooking, heat olive oil over medium heat in a large frying pan. Add onion slices in a single layer, and sauté until dark golden and tender, about 10 minutes. Set aside.

4. When rice has finished cooking, fluff with a fork, and turn out onto a serving platter. Pour oil and onions on top. Serve hot, garnished with lemon wedges.

- 1/2 cup dry chickpeas or 1 cup reduced-sodium, canned chickpeas
- 3 cups fat-free, low-sodium vegetable stock or water
- Salt, to taste
- Freshly ground pepper, to taste
- 1 1/2 cups basmati rice
- 1 tsp cumin
- 1/4 cup extra-virgin olive oil
- 2 large onions, quartered and sliced
- 1 lemon, sliced into 4 wedges

Healthy Living Tradition

To make variations of this recipe, lentils and other protein-rich legumes can be substituted for the chickpeas.

Exchanges/Choices	Calories	250	Sodium	60mg
2 Starch	Calories from Fat	70	**Total Carbohydrate**	40g
1 Vegetable	**Total Fat**	8.0g	Dietary Fiber	4g
1 1/2 Fat	Saturated Fat	1.1g	Sugars	4g
	Trans Fat	0.0g	**Protein**	5g
Serves 8	**Cholesterol**	0mg		
Serving Size: 1/2 cup				

Vegan dish

I believe that stuffed vegetables are one of the ultimate comfort foods. Whether I'm visiting friends and family in either Italy or Egypt, stuffed vegetables are usually part of the meal. Preparing stuffed vegetables is a labor of love whose results are both elegant and delicious. While preparing this recipe, you can make the stuffing in advance and then fill and bake before serving. Choose fresh, bright, in-season tomatoes for best results.

Rice and Herb Stuffed Tomatoes

1. Preheat oven to 350°F.

2. Place rice in a saucepan. Cover with water. Add salt, and bring to a boil over high heat. Cook, uncovered, for 12 minutes or until tender, but firm (*al dente*).

3. Meanwhile, cut the stems from the tomatoes. Carefully scoop out the insides, being sure not to tear the tomato skins. Place the tomatoes in a colander, and drain off excess liquid.

4. When rice is ready, drain it. Stir in olive oil and roasted red peppers. Chop the capers and the garlic together. Stir into rice mixture. Stir in dill, parsley, and mint.

3/4 cup Arborio rice
1/2 tsp sea or kosher salt
4 medium-sized beefsteak or vine-ripened tomatoes
1 Tbsp extra-virgin olive oil
2 jarred roasted red peppers, diced
2 Tbsp capers, drained
1 clove garlic, minced
1/4 cup fresh dill, finely chopped
1/4 cup fresh parsley, finely chopped
1/4 cup fresh mint, finely chopped

5. Stuff tomatoes with rice mixture, and place in a small baking dish. Bake for 20–30 minutes or until tomatoes are cooked through. Serve hot or at room temperature.

Healthy Living Tradition

Reducing your salt intake helps reduce water retention and is good for people who have high blood pressure. Mediterranean staple ingredients such as garlic, herbs, spices, and peppers make food taste better without adding more sodium.

Exchanges/Choices				
1 1/2 Starch	Calories	165	Sodium	465mg
1 Vegetable	Calories from Fat	35	Total Carbohydrate	30g
1/2 Fat	Total Fat	4.0g	Dietary Fiber	2g
	Saturated Fat	0.6g	Sugars	3g
	Trans Fat	0.0g	Protein	4g
Serves 4	Cholesterol	0mg		
Serving Size: 1 tomato				

Vegan dish

Artichokes and asparagus are a match made in heaven and are often paired in traditional Italian dishes. Asparagus and artichokes have many similarities. Both crops are native to the Mediterranean and grow best in a warm to slightly cool climate. In the kitchen, they can be used in soups, pastas, rice dishes, omelets, and salads.

Orzo with Lemon, Artichokes, and Asparagus

1. Bring a large pot of water to a boil over high heat. Add salt, reduce heat to medium, add orzo, and stir. Cook orzo until tender, but still *al dente*.

2. Bring a medium pot of water to a boil over high heat. Add asparagus, and cook until tender (about 5 minutes). Drain.

3. Drain orzo when it is done, and return to pot. Stir in asparagus, artichoke hearts, lemon juice, lemon zest, salt to taste, freshly ground pepper, and olive oil. Taste, and adjust seasoning, if necessary. Garnish with cheese, and serve hot.

- 1/4 tsp kosher salt
- 1 lb dry orzo pasta
- 1 lb trimmed asparagus, cut into 1-inch pieces (or frozen)
- 1 (14-oz) can artichoke hearts, drained and quartered
- 1/4 cup lemon juice
  Zest of 1 lemon
- 1/4 tsp freshly ground black pepper
- 2 Tbsp extra-virgin olive oil
- 1/4 cup Pecorino Romano cheese, for garnish

Healthy Living Tradition

The average American consumes only three servings of fruit and vegetables per day. Use this book for inspiration, and try doubling or tripling those servings by adding additional fruits and vegetables to recipes, even if they're not called for.

Exchanges/Choices				
2 1/2 Starch	**Calories**	255	**Sodium**	220mg
1 Vegetable	Calories from Fat	45	**Total Carbohydrate**	43g
1/2 Fat	**Total Fat**	5.0g	Dietary Fiber	3g
	Saturated Fat	1.1g	Sugars	6g
	Trans Fat	0.0g	**Protein**	9g
Serves 8	**Cholesterol**	5mg		
Serving Size: 1/2 cup				

Stuffed vegetables are an important part of the local diet in all Mediterranean countries. Popular stuffing ingredients range from rice to bread crumbs to bulgur. Bulgur is cracked wheat, which is high in fiber. To cook bulgur, boil the bulgur in double its amount of water (e.g., cook 1 cup bulgur in 2 cups water). When the water is absorbed, it's ready. It can be used in both sweet and savory recipes and is often used in cereals, stuffing, salads, and desserts. Note that many of the steps in this recipe can be done a day in advance.

Roasted Peppers Stuffed with Bulgur, Spinach, and Herbs

❋ Filfil Mashwi ma Burghol wa Khodar ❋

1. Preheat the oven to 425°F. Line a baking sheet with aluminum foil, and place peppers cut side down on it. Roast for 15 minutes, remove from oven, and turn peppers over. Roast for 15 minutes more. (This step can be done a day in advance.)

2. Make the filling by boiling 2 cups water in a medium saucepan. Remove from heat, and stir in bulgur. Cover, and let stand until bulgur is tender and water is absorbed (about 30 minutes). (This step can be done a day in advance.)

3. Meanwhile, heat olive oil in a large, wide skillet over medium heat. Sauté onion until tender, about 3 minutes. Add tomatoes, coriander, and cumin. Stir in spinach. Allow to cook about 3 minutes, stirring occasionally, until spinach is wilted.

3 green bell peppers, sliced in half lengthwise with ribs and seeds removed
1 cup bulgur
1 Tbsp extra-virgin olive oil
1 yellow onion, diced
1/4 cup diced canned low-sodium tomatoes
1 tsp ground coriander
1 tsp ground cumin
1/2 lb fresh spinach, chopped and stems trimmed
1/4 cup fresh parsley, finely chopped
1/4 cup fresh dill, finely chopped
1/4 cup fresh cilantro, finely chopped
2 Tbsp lemon juice
1 tsp salt
Freshly ground pepper, to taste

4. Mix in bulgur, parsley, dill, cilantro, lemon juice, salt, and freshly ground pepper to taste. Remove from heat. Divide bulgur mixture among pepper halves. (Peppers can be stuffed and stored a day in advance.)

5. Bake peppers about 20 minutes or until heated through. Serve warm or at room temperature.

Healthy Living Tradition

The Mediterranean region is famous for its wonderful herbs. By learning how to quickly and wisely use herbs, you'll be able to greatly enhance your culinary creations. Try washing and drying fresh herbs in a salad spinner. Next, store unused herbs wrapped in paper towels inside re-sealable plastic bags in your vegetable drawer. This way, they will be ready when you need them.

Exchanges/Choices		Calories	110	Sodium	420mg
1 Starch		Calories from Fat	25	**Total Carbohydrate**	20g
1 Vegetable		**Total Fat**	3.0g	Dietary Fiber	6g
1/2 Fat		Saturated Fat	0.4g	Sugars	3g
		Trans Fat	0.0g	**Protein**	4g
Serves 6		**Cholesterol**	0mg		
Serving Size: 1/2 pepper					

Vegan dish

This is a traditional first course offered in *trattorias* and homes throughout Italy. This recipe was developed as a way to use up abundant eggplants during harvest season. Norma is the name of the woman who had the wonderful idea of adding fried eggplant and sheep's milk cheese to a standard tomato sauce. This dish is so loved that other noteworthy acts are now referred to as *alla Norma*, meaning "successful" or "grandiose" in some parts of Sicily. This is one of my family's favorite dishes. I broil the eggplants instead of frying them.

Penne with Eggplant-Tomato Sauce

❋ *Penne alla Norma* ❋

1. Preheat broiler. Using a sharp knife, slice eggplant into 1/4-inch slices, and place on a baking sheet. Reserve 2 Tbsp olive oil, and brush the rest on the eggplant.

2. Broil for 5–7 minutes per side, until they are dark gold and cooked through. Set aside to cool. (This step can be done a day in advance.)

3. Heat reserved olive oil in a large saucepan over medium heat. Add garlic. Cook until it begins to release its aroma; do not allow garlic to turn color. Pour in tomatoes, and stir. Add crushed red pepper, basil, salt, and freshly ground pepper. Cover, reduce heat to low, and simmer for 20 minutes.

4. When eggplant is cool enough to handle, stack three slices together, and chop into dime-size pieces. Repeat until all eggplant is chopped.

5. Meanwhile, bring a gallon of water to a boil over high heat. Add pasta. Cook until *al dente*.

- 1 large (1 lb) eggplant
- 1/4 cup extra-virgin olive oil, divided
- 2 cloves garlic, minced
- 1 box or bottle (26 oz) strained tomatoes or tomato purée
  Pinch crushed red pepper flakes
- 6 fresh basil leaves, roughly torn
  Salt, to taste
  Freshly ground pepper, to taste
- 1/2 cup Pecorino Romano cheese
- 1 lb dried penne rigate

6. After sauce has cooked for 20 minutes, turn off heat, remove lid, and add eggplant pieces and cheese. Stir well. Cover, and simmer sauce over medium heat until pasta is done cooking (10–12 minutes).

7. Drain pasta. Toss in sauce to coat. Serve hot.

Healthy Living Tradition

Learning to make homemade tomato sauces and incorporating fresh vegetables will transform your meals into authentic, healthful Italian experiences.

Exchanges/Choices	Calories	335	Sodium	80mg
3 Starch	Calories from Fat	80	**Total Carbohydrate**	53g
2 Vegetable	**Total Fat**	9.0g	Dietary Fiber	5g
1 Fat	Saturated Fat	2.0g	Sugars	7g
	Trans Fat	0.0g	**Protein**	11g
Serves 8	**Cholesterol**	5mg		
Serving Size: 1/8 recipe				

One of the great advantages of living in Rome is being able to shop at the outdoor markets held daily or weekly in most neighborhoods. Fresh seasonal produce piled high provides inspiration for the city's chefs and home cooks alike. The Roman affinity for artichokes, garlic, and mint dates back to ancient times. This spaghetti dish is one of many typical Italian first-course pasta dishes that is tossed with fresh vegetables and herbs instead of ladled with a heavy sauce. Note that baby artichokes don't have the "choke" that needs to be removed from full-sized artichokes, so they are easier to clean.

Roman Spaghetti with Artichokes, Mint, and Garlic

1. *For fresh artichokes:* Soak the artichokes in water to clean. Drain and repeat until water is clear. Peel away the outer leaves of the bottom half of the artichokes. Cut off the top quarter of the artichoke (at this point, the artichoke should look like a flower, and the tough, dark leaves should be removed, leaving only lighter-colored tender leaves). If tough, dark green leaves remain, peel those off as well.

2. Squeeze out the lemon juice from the lemon into a bowl of water. Then drop the artichokes into the water to prevent discoloration.

3. Bring a large pot of water to a boil, and add cleaned artichokes. Bring to boil over high heat. Reduce heat to medium low, and simmer 15–20 minutes or until tender. Drain artichokes, and set aside.

24 **baby artichokes, peeled and trimmed, or 2 cans reduced-sodium artichokes, drained**
   Juice of 1 lemon (only if using fresh artichokes)
1 **lb whole-wheat spaghetti**
3 **Tbsp extra-virgin olive oil**
4 **cloves garlic, minced**
1/2 **tsp sea or kosher salt**
1/8 **tsp freshly ground black pepper**
1 **cup fresh mint, finely chopped**
   Pinch crushed red chili flakes

4. Prepare spaghetti according to package directions until *al dente*. Drain.

5. Meanwhile, heat olive oil in a large, wide skillet over medium heat. When oil coats the bottom of the pan and begins to release its aroma, add garlic. Reduce heat to low. Cook garlic just until it begins to release its aroma, before it turns color. Add artichokes, salt, and pepper, and fry for a minute on each side until golden. Add pasta, mint, and red pepper flakes to the skillet, and turn to coat. Serve warm.

Healthy Living Tradition

Check with your local farmers' markets to find out when fresh artichokes are available in your area. You can cook many at a time, drain them, and allow them to cool. Then freeze them in plastic freezer bags in serving-size portions, so you'll always have them on hand.

Exchanges/Choices		Calories	310	Sodium	280mg
2 1/2 Starch		Calories from Fat	55	**Total Carbohydrate**	53g
2 Vegetable		**Total Fat**	6.0g	Dietary Fiber	14g
1 Fat		Saturated Fat	0.9g	Sugars	2g
		Trans Fat	0.0g	**Protein**	12g
Serves 8		**Cholesterol**	0mg		
Serving Size: about 1 cup					

Saffron is the world's most expensive spice. It is cultivated from the stigmas of the crocus flower in fall. Its English name is derived from the plural of the feminine form of the Arabic word for "yellow," *saffra*. Saffron provides a bright yellow color and unique flavor to drinks, savories, and sweets. In traditional Mediterranean medicine, saffron is used to increase energy, suppress coughs, rejuvenate the heart, and ease labor pains.

Saffron Couscous

1. Bring 1 cup water and saffron to a boil, uncovered, in a medium saucepan with a lid. When water is boiling, remove pan from heat, and add couscous. Mix well, cover pan with lid, and let stand for 5–10 minutes. Remove lid. Add olive oil. Stir, add salt, and fluff with a fork. Spoon couscous onto a large serving platter. Sprinkle roasted almonds on top. Serve immediately.

1	tsp saffron
1 1/4	cups couscous
1	Tbsp extra-virgin olive oil
	Salt, to taste
1/4	cup roasted almonds, slivered

Healthy Living Tradition

Across the Mediterranean region, people often gather to make traditional dishes. Cooking communally is a healthful activity because it encourages homemade food and reinforces human bonding. Invent new ways for your friends and family to congregate and cook healthy meals together whenever possible.

Exchanges/Choices	Calories	200	Sodium	5mg
2 Starch	Calories from Fat	45	**Total Carbohydrate**	32g
1 Fat	**Total Fat**	5.0g	Dietary Fiber	2g
	Saturated Fat	0.6g	Sugars	1g
Serves 5	Trans Fat	0.0g	**Protein**	6g
Serving Size: 1/2 cup	**Cholesterol**	0mg		

Vegan dish

Quick-cooking couscous and low-sodium canned beans are must-haves in a Mediterranean pantry. By tossing them together with fresh herbs and vegetables, you can have a delicious dish in less than 15 minutes! If you don't have fresh herbs on hand, simply add a teaspoon of your favorite dried herbs or spice instead.

Couscous with Tomatoes, Black Beans, and Herbs

1. Bring 1 cup water to a boil in a medium saucepan. Stir in olive oil and couscous, remove from heat, and cover tightly. Fluff with a fork to separate granules. Add beans, tomatoes, salt, pepper, cilantro, parsley, and mint. Serve warm.

1	Tbsp extra-virgin olive oil
1 1/4	cups couscous
1	(15-oz) can low-sodium black beans, rinsed and drained
10	cherry tomatoes, quartered
1/4	tsp salt
	Pinch black pepper
1/4	cup fresh cilantro, finely chopped
1/4	cup parsley, finely chopped
1/4	cup mint, finely chopped

Healthy Living Tradition

In addition to cooking quickly, couscous is also a great source of phosphorus and potassium. Use recipes like this one on busy nights instead of ordering in or eating out.

Exchanges/Choices		Calories	140	Sodium	70mg
1 1/2 Starch		Calories from Fat	20	Total Carbohydrate	25g
		Total Fat	2.0g	Dietary Fiber	3g
Serves 9		Saturated Fat	0.3g	Sugars	1g
Serving Size: 1/2 cup		Trans Fat	0.0g	Protein	5g
		Cholesterol	0mg		
Vegan dish					

Magical Mediterranean Mains

From French classics like *Tarragon Supreme of Chicken with Mushrooms* (p. 103) to *Valencian Seafood Paella* (p. 130) and *Israeli Orange and Honey-Glazed Chicken with Almonds* (p. 94), Mediterranean-style main dishes are delicious escapes from culinary boredom. Poultry, seafood, beans, legumes, and vegetables are common denominators in the main dishes of this region. The use of herbs, citrus, and spices, as well as cooking and serving methods, however, tend to be country or culture specific.

Since ancient times, the geography and climates of the various countries surrounding the Mediterranean Sea ensured the presence of fertile lands capable of cultivating large amounts of crops. Farmers, fisherman, and shepherds provided ingredients to housewives and artisans, who created the healthful cuisine that is the foundation of the Mediterranean diet today.

In the southern European countries of France, Spain, Portugal, and Italy, main courses usually contain a small portion of lean meat, seafood, or poultry; cooked vegetables and legumes; and vegetable-based sauces. This is because until refrigeration was invented, people could not conserve foods for long periods of time. Dried staples could only be supplemented by fresh, in-season or preserved produce.

Even though major supermarket chains now stock large varieties of produce year-round, freshness is still the key component in Mediterranean-style cooking. Seasonal cuisine is culturally and nutritionally valued. In addition to being less expensive, seasonal, local produce requires less transportation, making it safer for the environment, better tasting, and better for us.

Southern European countries have made eating seasonally an art form. During the spring, new baby vegetables, asparagus, artichokes, fennel, and young animals, like sheep and veal, are popular choices.

During the summer, fresh local herbs, market produce, and seafood take center stage. During the fall, apples, pears, broccoli, squash, chestnuts, and mushrooms are eaten. In the winter, dried fruits, preserved vegetables and pickles, root vegetables (such as potatoes, dried beans, and legumes), and grains are main components of the Mediterranean diet. Dairy products—such as cow, sheep, and goat's milk; yogurt and cheeses; and eggs—are eaten year-round.

In the North African, Greek, and Middle Eastern parts of the Mediterranean, the seasons tend to be less pronounced than in southern Europe. Hot, dry weather lasts for longer periods, making fresh produce available longer. In these areas, the same type of food is eaten year-round. Growing cycles and harvest times in each geographic area determine what is eaten each month. Although supermarkets exist in these areas, too, most people still prefer fresh, local produce. A drive down any suburban street or visit to any urban marketplace will reveal mounds of ripe, plump, perfect produce, making it difficult to justify paying for expensive, out-of-season foods.

In North Africa and the Middle East, fresh fruit juices are enjoyed year-round. Fresh oranges may be abundant in January and February, and kiwi and pomegranates in March. Stuffed vegetables are also prepared year-round. In the winter, stuffed cabbage is enjoyed; in the spring, *Stuffed Vine Leaves (p. 34)*; in summer, stuffed baby eggplant; and in fall, stuffed zucchini. As seasons overlap, so do the foods prepared.

Throughout this part of the Mediterranean, hot soups, stews, and teas are served on cold nights and hot days alike. Main dishes tend to be grilled or roasted seafood, poultry, or meat, served with vegetables, or they can be vegetable-based stews and casseroles that include smaller amounts of meat. Because meat historically has been scarce in Greece, North Africa, and the Middle East, it is more prized. The main dish is the crescendo around which the entire meal revolves. Unless they are vegetarians, Greek, North African, and Middle Eastern hosts will always offer meat dishes when entertaining guests to honor them. Doing this honors them. The daily diets, however, rely heavily on produce, beans, legumes, grains, and seafood. Rich dairy products, such as thick whole milk, sheep's and goat's yogurt, cheeses, and eggs, are also important staples.

In addition to the numerous agricultural advantages to living in the Mediterranean, the region's rich heritage of power, politics, trade, and commerce elevated each country's cooking standards. The kitchens of pharaohs, emperors, kings, and sultans mandated that food be not only tasty and healthy, but also a visual demonstration of high social status. Even more, religious traditions contributed unique celebratory and fasting foods to each culture.

The ancient civilizations of Egypt, Greece, and Rome spread new and prestigious culinary trends throughout the region. Egyptian papyri from 2800 BCE describe extensive use of spices only 200 years after the first accounts of spices were recorded in China. Fava beans, such as those used in the *Fava Bean Purée* (p. 36), have actually been used since those past ages. In Egypt, Old Kingdom (2700–2600 BCE) tomb scenes depict bread being shaped and produced in mass quantities. Ramses II's tomb contains pictures of elegant pastries, cakes, and pies being made in bakeries that catered to royalty. During antiquity, the city of Alexandria, Egypt, and its legendary library were considered the center of learning for the entire Mediterranean region. At one time, the Egyptian empire spanned from Sudan in the south to Lebanon in the north. For this reason as well as geographic ones, the countries of northeast Africa and the Levantine continue to have many dishes in common today.

The Greeks also came to Egypt in pursuit of knowledge. They employed scribes to record their findings in Egypt, and those texts were distributed throughout the Mediterranean. The first Roman epicurean, Apicius, wrote accounts of bread from Alexandria in his cookbook, *On Cooking.* Roman emperors sent fleets to the shores of North Africa to obtain their superior seafood, spices, sugar, wheat, and other supplies. It is out of this ancient tradition of trade and exchange that culinary commonalities in the Mediterranean grew and continue to flourish today.

There are, however, unique food traditions in the Mediterranean region that are country specific. European nobility would often marry into foreign courts to increase the geographic boundaries of their power. In addition to wedding vows, recipes were exchanged, and the bride's culinary contributions would often become integral parts of the cuisine of her adopted homeland. In the countries of North Africa and the Middle East, both kings and sultans created competing empires and dynasties. Often, ruling parties would seek to distinguish themselves as superior by outdoing one another with sophisticated and elaborate recipes.

In Turkey, thousands of chefs worked in the kitchens of the Topkapi Palace at the same time. Each chef specialized in one dish alone and had 100 understudies to ensure that the culinary heritage was carried on. *Circassian Chicken and Lettuce* (p. 89) and *Stuffed Vine Leaves (p. 34)* were born out of the lavish Turkish cooking styles. During the reign of Sultan al Nasir Muhammad in Egypt, the kitchens of the Cairo citadel produced more than 25,000 tons of food per day. A typical banquet consisted of thousands of animals and tons of sugar for desserts and sorbets. The Abassid dynasty in Iraq viewed cuisine as an art form and served extravagant recipes for the time. Later, the rivaling Ummayad dynasty in southern Spain and Morocco employed members of the Abassid courts in order to surpass them in creating culinary masterpieces. Centuries later, these elegant court recipes continue to be recreated by home cooks and professional chefs alike. By combining simple, fresh ingredients with time-honored traditions and straightforward cooking styles, the cultures of the Mediterranean have created some of the world's best dishes. This book contains simple, easy-to-recreate versions that will guarantee pleasure and success each time you cook and eat them.

The Spirit in Which Food Is Offered

In cities, towns, and villages dotting the Mediterranean coastline, most main dishes are served family style at home. Restaurant dining is not an important part of local cultures. Many people pride themselves on never having to go to a restaurant. The majority of the people highly value home cooking and recognize the importance of eating with their families. Gathering for meals is a part of daily life in most areas in the region. It is believed that the spirit in which food is offered is as important as the food itself. Therefore, delicious, healthy, homemade cuisine should be made by and shared with loved ones.

The inhabitants of the island of Sardinia, off of Italy's west coast, have been found to live healthier, longer lives than people of other cultures. In addition to a traditional Mediterranean diet, researchers found that sitting down for a homemade family meal was one of the contributing factors for the optimal health experienced by Sardinians. Communal meals were also found to promote feelings of support and stability, which help prevent depression and other psychological problems.

To achieve the maximum benefits of the Mediterranean diet, one must not only cook Mediterranean recipes, but also adopt the belief that giving, receiving, and enjoying food with others is a necessity, not a luxury. Even in today's busy modern life, we can find many occasions to eat with family and friends. Here are some tips to make the transformation easy:

1. Plan your meals. Plan meals on a weekly basis. Decide which dishes you have time to prepare. Make a grocery list and a schedule of when you will prepare which dishes.

2. Take your schedule into consideration. On days when you have an hour to cook, try preparing two quick main dishes, one to eat that day and one to keep for a day when you don't have time to cook.

3. Involve family members in the process. Post a schedule on the refrigerator and delegate tasks. One person can make the salad, another can do prep work, etc.

4. Start with easy recipes. Save elaborate meals for holidays and special occasions.

5. Have cooking/baking parties with friends and relatives. Invite people over to cook meals. Once you've finished, sit down and enjoy the fruits of your labor.

6. Start a theme night. If you have trouble getting everyone to sit down and eat together, start a theme night. One night a week, pick a theme, such as a favorite vacation spot, a place your children are studying in school, or a place you would like to visit. Prepare a favorite dish associated with that theme, and follow up with an activity that ties in with the theme.

7. Start a journal. Keep a journal and record your differences in eating styles, emotions, and physical feelings after eating homemade food versus prepared food. Write down how you felt eating by yourself or with family and friends. People in the Mediterranean region are very tuned in to their eating process. It's a major topic of conversation, and people think about it all day. In the U.S., we tend to think of mealtime as something we *have* to do, instead of something we *want* to do. Use your journal to write down the benefits of home cooking and eating communally. Periodically read the journal to reinforce the importance of your Mediterranean dining trends.

Shwarma **is the rotisserie-cooked meat that is shaved off and piled high in sandwiches all** over the Middle East. Traditionally, the meat is threaded with layers of fat, topped with tomatoes and/or peppers, and left to cook slowly for hours. This recipe enables you to enjoy this popular street food at home, saving time and calories. Remember to marinate the chicken for 24 hours before preparing this recipe. Serve with *Tahini Sauce* (p. 279) and pickled vegetables.

Chicken Pita Sandwiches

❋ *Shwarma bil Dajaj* ❋

1. Combine all ingredients, except pita bread, in a large shallow bowl or dish. Stir to mix well and coat chicken. Cover with foil and place in refrigerator for 24 hours.

2. After chicken has marinated for 24 hours, preheat oven to 425°F. Remove chicken from refrigerator. Drain well. Spread chicken in a single layer on a baking sheet. Bake on the lower rack of the oven for 25 minutes, turning once. Taste, and adjust seasonings if necessary. Remove from oven. Top pitas with chicken mixture. Fold in half to serve like a taco. Serve on a platter with small bowls of hot sauce, tahini sauce, and pickles.

1 **lb boneless, skinless chicken breasts (sliced into 1/2-inch-long pieces)**
1 **tsp salt**
1 **tsp freshly ground pepper**
Dash chili powder
1 **tsp cumin**
1 **tsp paprika**
Juice and zest of 1 lemon
1/8 **cup white vinegar**
2 **Tbsp olive oil**
5 **cloves garlic, chopped**
2 **medium onions, chopped**
4 **pieces** Whole-Wheat Pita Bread **(p. 258)**

Healthy Living Tradition

Leftover roasted chicken can be used to make these delicious sandwiches in only a few moments. Heat 1 Tbsp olive oil in a large skillet. Add diced green pepper, chopped yellow onion, and a diced tomato. Cook over medium-high heat until vegetables are tender. Add shredded leftover meat, cumin, coriander, salt, and pepper. Stuff meat in pita pockets, and serve warm.

Exchanges/Choices		Calories	280	Sodium	470mg
1 1/2 Starch		Calories from Fat	65	**Total Carbohydrate**	24g
4 Lean Meat		**Total Fat**	7.0g	Dietary Fiber	2g
		Saturated Fat	1.4g	Sugars	1g
Serves 4		Trans Fat	0.0g	**Protein**	28g
Serving Size: 1 pita + 4 oz filling		**Cholesterol**	65mg		

Souvlakia **is the Greek word for "kabobs."** They can be made with chicken, veal, or beef. Keep in mind that they need to be marinated for at least 30 minutes to a maximum of overnight. You will need skewers to make the kabobs. If you are using wooden skewers, soak them in water for 30 minutes while the meat is marinating to prevent them from burning. Serve with *Whole-Wheat Pita Bread* (p. 258) and *Cucumber, Yogurt, and Dill Salad* (p. 32).

Greek Chicken Souvlaki

❋ **Souvlaki** ❋

1. Combine lemon juice, garlic, salt, pepper, olive oil, and parsley in a large shallow dish. Stir to combine. Add chicken. Turn to coat and cover. Marinate for at least 30 minutes to overnight.

2. When chicken has finished marinating, scrape off excess marinade. Loosely skewer meat on skewers, about 1/4 lb of meat per skewer.

1/2	**cup fresh lemon juice**
6	**cloves garlic, minced**
1	**tsp salt**
	Freshly ground pepper, to taste
2	**Tbsp extra-virgin olive oil**
4	**Tbsp fresh parsley**
1	**lb chicken breast cubes**

3. Heat a grill over medium-high heat. Place skewers on grill, and cook for 2–3 minutes, until bottoms are seared. Using potholders or oven mitts, rotate skewers. Continue grilling and rotating every 3 minutes, until desired level of doneness is reached. If using a grill pan, 20 minutes should produce well-done meat. When done, remove from heat and wrap in foil. Let stand 5 minutes before eating.

Healthy Living Tradition

Citrus juice, olive oil, garlic, and fresh herbs make fantastic Mediterranean marinades that can be used for all kinds of meats, poultry, seafood, and vegetables. Try this easy and nutritious version instead of store-bought varieties, which are full of additives.

Exchanges/Choices		Calories	165	Sodium	355mg
3 Lean Meat		Calories from Fat	55	**Total Carbohydrate**	2g
1/2 Fat		**Total Fat**	6.0g	Dietary Fiber	0g
		Saturated Fat	1.2g	Sugars	0g
Serves 4		Trans Fat	0.0g	**Protein**	24g
Serving Size: 1 skewer		**Cholesterol**	65mg		

This simple chicken breast recipe contains a topping reminiscent of Caprese salad. The word *"Caprese"* describes anything native to the Italian island of Capri, located off the coastline near Naples. Capri is famous for its picture-perfect location, delicious food, and enormous lemons, which are grown at the foot of Mount Vesuvius.

Caprese-Style Chicken Breasts
❋ *Petti di Pollo alla Caprese* ❋

1. Season chicken with salt and pepper. Heat olive oil in a large, wide, oven-proof skillet over medium heat. Add garlic and chicken. Cook chicken 5 minutes per side, turning once, or until no longer pink.

2. Sprinkle crushed red chili flakes over the chicken, and squeeze lemon juice over the top. Preheat broiler.

3. Top each piece of chicken with 4 tomato slices and 1/4 of the mozzarella. Place under broiler, and broil until cheese is golden (about 3 minutes).

4. Remove from oven, and top with fresh basil. Serve with 1 cup cooked broccoli.

2 boneless, skinless chicken breasts (8 oz each), sliced in half crosswise, yielding 4 (4-oz) pieces
1/2 tsp salt
Freshly ground pepper, to taste
1 Tbsp extra-virgin olive oil
4 cloves garlic, minced
Pinch crushed red chili flakes
1/4 cup freshly squeezed lemon juice
2 Roma tomatoes, sliced into 8 slices each
2 oz part-skim mozzarella, shredded
1/4 cup fresh basil, finely chopped
4 cups cooked broccoli

Healthy Living Tradition

Scaloppine—or thinly sliced pieces of veal, beef, chicken, or turkey, which are used in this recipe—is a favorite second course among Italians. It is the perfect choice for weeknight dinners because it cooks in a few minutes. Scaloppine can be topped with lemon juice or quick pan sauces. Thinly sliced pieces of meat and poultry are also great for entertaining because they are not too filling and allow guests to savor different courses and flavors at one meal.

Exchanges/Choices				
2 Vegetable	Calories	250	Sodium	480mg
4 Lean Meat	Calories from Fat	80	**Total Carbohydrate**	12g
1/2 Fat	**Total Fat**	9.0g	Dietary Fiber	5g
	Saturated Fat	2.7g	Sugars	3g
	Trans Fat	0.0g	**Protein**	33g
Serves 4	**Cholesterol**	75mg		
Serving Size: 1 piece chicken breast				

Chicken, Dijon-based sauce, and zucchini are a classic French combination. This recipe is simple enough to make any time, yet will also impress guests.

Dijon-Glazed Chicken Breasts with Zucchini

❋ *Escalope de Poulet avec la Sauce Dijonaise et Courgettes* ❋

1. Mix flour, salt, and pepper together in a large shallow bowl. Lightly coat each chicken breast, and set aside.

2. Heat olive oil over medium heat in a large, wide skillet. Add chicken. Cook for 5 minutes on each side or until brown, turning once. Pour stock over chicken. Arrange zucchini slices around chicken, so that they are covered by the stock. Bring mixture to a boil. Reduce heat to low, cover, and simmer for 10–12 minutes or until chicken and zucchini are cooked through.

3. With a slotted spoon, remove chicken and zucchini and place on a serving platter. Add mustard to remaining stock in the pan, and whisk to incorporate. Increase heat to high. Cook for a few minutes or until sauce has thickened and barely coats the bottom of pan. Pour sauce over chicken and zucchini. Sprinkle fresh parsley over the top.

- **1/4 cup all-purpose flour**
- **1/2 tsp salt**
  Freshly ground pepper, to taste
- **2 boneless, skinless chicken breasts (8 oz each), sliced in half widthwise into 4 (4-oz) pieces**
- **1 Tbsp extra-virgin olive oil**
- **2 cups fat-free, low-sodium chicken or vegetable stock**
- **3 zucchini (about 6 oz each), cut into thin slices**
- **2 Tbsp Dijon mustard**
- **1/4 cup fresh Italian parsley, finely chopped**

Healthy Living Tradition

Although it is botanically considered a fruit, zucchini is treated as a vegetable in culinary uses. It is low in calories, high in vitamin C, and full of antioxidants, making it a wonderful staple in Mediterranean households.

Exchanges/Choices		Calories	225	Sodium	585mg
1/2 Starch • 1 Vegetable		Calories from Fat	65	**Total Carbohydrate**	12g
3 Lean Meat • 1/2 Fat		**Total Fat**	7.0g	Dietary Fiber	2g
		Saturated Fat	1.4g	Sugars	3g
Serves 4		Trans Fat	0.0g	**Protein**	28g
Serving Size: 1 piece chicken,		**Cholesterol**	70mg		
2 Tbsp sauce, and 1/2 cup zucchini					

During the late 16th century, King Henry IV of France declared that every working family in his kingdom would have a chicken in every pot on Sunday. Since then, roasted chicken has become a classic Sunday dish in France. Let local availability and taste determine which vegetables to include in this dish. Potatoes, carrots, and cherry tomatoes or fennel, chestnuts, and shallots also make great additions.

French Roasted Chicken with Green Beans

1. Preheat oven to 425°F. Place chicken in a roasting pan. Drizzle olive oil over the chicken, turning to make sure that both the pan and chicken are coated. Season with salt, pepper, and *Herbes de Provence* by rubbing them into the top and sides of the chicken. Place garlic and a lemon half inside the chicken cavity. Squeeze remaining juice from the other lemon half over the chicken.

2. Bake, uncovered, for 45 minutes. Carefully (oil can splatter) remove chicken from the oven, and scatter green beans around the edges. Turn green beans in olive oil to coat. Season with lemon zest and lemon juice. Turn again to coat well.

3. Return to oven, and bake for another 45 minutes or until chicken is done and green beans are tender. (Chicken is done when clear juices run from the thickest part of the thigh after being pierced with a fork.) Cover chicken. Wait 10 minutes before carving. Discard garlic and lemon from cavity. Remove chicken skin before serving.

1   **whole chicken (3.5 lb), cleaned and rinsed well**
1/4   **cup extra-virgin olive oil**
1   **tsp French sea salt**
    Freshly ground pepper, to taste
1   **Tbsp Herbes de Provence (p. 277)**
1   **head garlic, stem sliced off, left intact**
2   **lemons, divided (1 sliced in half, 1 zested and juiced)**
1   **lb green beans, trimmed**

Healthy Living Tradition

Plan a casual gathering around a simple, healthful Mediterranean meal with main courses like this one and rediscover the pleasure of entertaining at home.

Exchanges/Choices		Calories	170	Sodium	205mg
1 Vegetable		Calories from Fat	70	**Total Carbohydrate**	4g
3 Lean Meat		**Total Fat**	8.0g	Dietary Fiber	2g
1/2 Fat		Saturated Fat	1.8g	Sugars	1g
		Trans Fat	0.0g	**Protein**	19g
Serves 8		**Cholesterol**	55mg		
Serving Size: 3 oz chicken + 1/2 cup green beans					

This is a quick and healthy "modern" version of a classic Turkish dish, which is similar to chicken salad. The original version calls for a whole chicken, which is then cut up and used to make a home-made stock. My Turkish friends Aysel Yuksel and Zehra Yargici shared this dish with me. Serve it cold or at room temperature, in lettuce cups at a buffet, as an appetizer, or for lunch.

Circassian Chicken and Lettuce

❋ Çerkes Tavuğu ❋

1. Place chicken breasts in a stockpot, cover with stock, and add pepper. Bring to a boil over high heat, reduce heat to medium low, and cook for 30 minutes. Remove scum with a slotted spoon when it appears. When chicken is cooked through, remove it from liquid with a slotted spoon, and strain liquid into another bowl or container.

2. Place bread, walnuts, garlic, 1 cup reserved stock, and milk in a food processor or blender. Pulse on and off to form a sauce.

3. When chicken is cool enough to handle, shred it into bite-size pieces. Add it to the sauce.

4. Combine corn oil and paprika in a small bowl.

5. Transfer chicken to a serving plate, flatten slightly, and make a well in the center. Pour oil-paprika mixture into the center, and serve with lettuce leaves or bread.

- **3 lb boneless, skinless chicken breasts**
- **3 cups fat-free, low-sodium chicken stock**
- **1/4 tsp freshly ground black pepper**
- **3 slices day-old bread, cubed**
- **1 cup walnuts, ground**
- **1 clove garlic, chopped**
- **1/2 cup nonfat milk**
- **1 Tbsp corn oil**
- **1 tsp paprika**

Healthy Living Tradition

In some parts of the Middle East, some believe that walnuts improve brain function! Regardless of whether that's true, they are a great source of heart-healthy polyunsaturated fat.

Exchanges/Choices	Calories	270	Total Carbohydrate	6g
1/2 Carbohydrate	Calories from Fat	115	Dietary Fiber	1g
4 Lean Meat	**Total Fat**	13.0g	Sugars	1g
1 Fat	Saturated Fat	1.9g	**Protein**	32g
	Trans Fat	0.0g		
Serves 10	**Cholesterol**	80mg		
Serving Size: about 1/2 cup	**Sodium**	165mg		

Versions of this dish date back to the 9th century. Preserved lemons are enjoyed throughout North Africa. They can be eaten with a meal, like pickles, or added to soups, stews, and meat recipes. This surprisingly simple chicken dish is stewed with spices and preserved lemons on top of the stove rather than in the oven. The chicken is moist, tender, and full of fruity and smoky Moroccan flavor.

Moroccan Chicken with Preserved Lemons

1. Heat oil in a large pot over medium heat. Add onions, and sauté until tender (about 5 minutes). Add garlic, and stir. Add whole chicken, and brown on all sides. When chicken is browned, add ginger, paprika, cumin, and saffron. Cover with stock, and bring to a boil. If stock does not cover chicken, add some water. Add salt, pepper, lemons, and olives. Stir, reduce heat to medium low, and cover the pot. Simmer for 1 hour.

2. When chicken is cooked through, remove it, and set it on a carving board. Cover it with foil, and let rest for 10 minutes.

3. Keep the pot with the sauce on the stove. Increase the temperature to high. Allow sauce to boil while chicken rests.

4. After chicken has rested, remove the skin and carve. Arrange meat on a serving platter. Ladle half of the sauce over the chicken. Reserve remaining half of the sauce. Garnish with chopped cilantro. Serve hot.

1	Tbsp extra-virgin olive oil
2	medium onions, sliced
2	cloves garlic, minced
1	whole chicken (4 lb)
1	tsp ground ginger
1	tsp paprika
1	tsp cumin
	Pinch saffron threads
6	cups fat-free, low-sodium chicken stock
1/4	tsp salt
1/4	tsp freshly ground pepper
4	preserved lemons or 1 fresh lemon, quartered
1/4	cup black olives, pitted
1/4	cup chopped fresh cilantro

Healthy Living Tradition

This recipe yields a lot more sauce than needed to dress the chicken. Save the remaining sauce in the freezer. The next time you are going to make this recipe, simply defrost the sauce, heat it up on the stove, add the chicken, and allow it to simmer until it is ready. Enjoy the same great taste with a lot less work.

Exchanges/Choices	Calories	165	Sodium	310mg
3 Lean Meat	Calories from Fat	65	Total Carbohydrate	4g
1/2 Fat	**Total Fat**	7.0g	Dietary Fiber	1g
	Saturated Fat	1.6g	Sugars	1g
Serves 8	Trans Fat	0.0g	**Protein**	22g
Serving Size: 4 oz chicken	**Cholesterol**	65mg		

I first experienced this exquisite dish at a restaurant called Kazan's in northern Virginia. It consists of tender, moist chicken morsels and crisp, chewy, bread croutons swimming in a light oregano-infused tomato sauce. It is served over a bed of cooling yogurt. The combination of flavors, tastes, and textures quickly made it one of my favorite dishes. In this version, I have replaced the butter with olive oil and the whole-milk yogurt with low-fat, but the applications and flavors are still the same. Note that the yogurt in this recipe needs to be drained overnight.

Turkish Chicken with Tomato Sauce and Yogurt

1. Place a colander inside a bowl. Add yogurt. Set in the refrigerator for 6 hours or overnight.

2. Heat oil in a large saucepan over medium heat. Add chicken. Brown on all sides (about 5 minutes total). Add tomatoes, 1 cup water, paprika, oregano, salt, and pepper. Stir to combine. Increase heat to high, and bring to a boil, uncovered. Reduce heat to low, cover, and simmer for 1–1 1/2 hours or until chicken is tender.

3. Meanwhile, preheat the oven to 200°F. Toast pita for 5–10 minutes per side or until lightly golden.

4. When chicken is cooked through, stir in pita pieces and remove from heat. Spread drained yogurt on the bottom of a serving platter. Top with chicken stew mixture. Serve hot.

- **2 cups** low-fat plain yogurt, drained overnight
- **2 Tbsp** extra-virgin olive oil
- **1 1/2 lb** boneless, skinless chicken breast, cut into 1-inch cubes
- **1 cup** chopped or diced low-sodium canned tomatoes
- **1 tsp** sweet paprika
- **1 Tbsp** freshly chopped oregano or **1/2 tsp** dried oregano
- **1/2 tsp** kosher salt
- **1/4 tsp** freshly ground black pepper
- **1** pita bread, cut into 1/2-inch cubes

Healthy Living Tradition

Tomatoes are a wonderful source of important nutrients. When fresh tomatoes are not in season, rely on recipes with tomato-based sauces to get the nutrients you need.

Exchanges/Choices			
1/2 Starch • 1/2 Fat-Free Milk			
1 Vegetable • 5 Lean Meat			
1/2 Fat			

Calories	370	**Sodium**	500mg
Calories from Fat	115	**Total Carbohydrate**	19g
Total Fat	13.0g	Dietary Fiber	2g
Saturated Fat	3.0g	Sugars	5g
Trans Fat	0.0g	**Protein**	44g
Cholesterol	105mg		

Serves 4
Serving Size: 1/2 cup stew + 1/4 cup yogurt

Throughout the Middle East, sauces made with tahini are served to accompany kabobs. In this recipe, chicken morsels are marinated in tahini to give them additional flavor and protein. The glaze can be served beside or on top of the chicken. This recipe can be made on the grill or under the broiler. Flat, metal skewers are the easiest to use because the flat shape prevents the chicken pieces from turning around during cooking and they don't need soaking. Wooden skewers need to be soaked in water for at least 30 minutes before use to prevent burning.

Sesame-Coated Chicken Kabobs with Raspberry-Mustard Glaze

1. In a large bowl, combine tahini, lemon juice, and garlic. Whisk together with a fork. Continue whisking, and stir in 1/4 cup water a little at a time to form a smooth dressing. Add salt, pepper, and chili flakes. Stir to combine.

2. Rinse chicken pieces, and add to tahini sauce. Turn to coat. Marinate, covered, for 1 hour at room temperature or overnight in the refrigerator.

3. Preheat broiler, grill, or grill pan. Evenly thread chicken pieces onto six skewers. Discard leftover marinade. Grill chicken, turning frequently, until golden brown on the outside and cooked through on the inside (about 20 minutes).

1/3 cup tahini (sesame paste)
     Juice of 1/2 lemon
  2 cloves garlic, minced
1/8 tsp salt
     Dash freshly ground pepper
     Dash crushed red chili flakes, if desired
  2 lb boneless, skinless chicken breasts, cubed
  2 tsp Dijon mustard
  2 tsp honey
2/3 cup mashed fresh or frozen raspberries with juice
  2 Tbsp canola oil
  1 head romaine lettuce, cored and chopped into bite-size pieces

4. Make dressing by combining mustard, honey, and mashed raspberries with juice in a small bowl. Whisk in canola oil to form a smooth glaze. Place in a small serving bowl. Line the bottom of a serving platter with lettuce. Lay chicken pieces on top and brush with glaze. Serve warm.

Healthy Living Tradition

Packaged salad dressings are full of chemicals, preservatives, and unnecessary ingredients. Take a tip from Mediterranean kitchens: serve salads with extra-virgin olive oil, lemon juice, lime juice, or vinegar. Using Dijon mustard and raspberries (as in this recipe) will give you a thicker consistency and additional flavor without adding a lot of calories or fat.

Exchanges/Choices	Calories		Sodium	
1/2 Carbohydrate	Calories from Fat	110	Total Carbohydrate	7g
5 Lean Meat	**Total Fat**	12.0g	Dietary Fiber	3g
1/2 Fat	Saturated Fat	1.9g	Sugars	3g
	Trans Fat	0.0g	**Protein**	34g
Serves 6	**Cholesterol**	90mg		
Serving Size: 3–4 oz chicken				

Calories 275

This sensational sweet and sour chicken dish hails from Israel and is accompanied by fragrant basmati rice. Serve with *Bean, Lentil, and Spinach Skillet* (p. 164) and *Carrot, Date, and Orange Salad* (p. 176) and you'll have a healthful Middle Eastern feast.

Israeli Orange and Honey-Glazed Chicken with Almonds

1. Preheat oven to 425°F. Place honey in a small saucepan. Heat over low heat until fluid; reserve.

2. Place chicken in a roasting pan greased with olive oil. Put garlic in the chicken cavity. Pour warm honey over the top. Pour orange juice around the base of the pan, and season chicken with salt and pepper. Roast for about 1 hour and 45 minutes (basting every 20 minutes) or until juices run clear from the thigh when pierced. (If blood comes out, the chicken is not done).

3. After the chicken has been roasting for 1 hour, begin preparing the rice. Combine olive oil, rice, boiling water, turmeric, cinnamon, ginger, and salt to taste over high heat. Cook, uncovered, until all of the water is absorbed. Stir in raisins, lower the heat to the lowest level possible, and cover tightly. Cook for 10 minutes, turn off heat, and let stand for 10 minutes.

Chicken

- 1 **Tbsp honey**
- 1 **whole roasting chicken (3 1/2 lb), rinsed, skin and giblets removed, and dried**
- 1 **tsp extra-virgin olive oil**
- 2 **cloves garlic**
- 2 **oranges, juiced**
- 1/2 **tsp kosher salt**
- 1/4 **tsp freshly ground pepper**

Rice

- 1 **Tbsp extra-virgin olive oil**
- 1 **cup basmati rice, soaked in water for 20 minutes and drained**
- 1 3/4 **cups boiling water**
- 1 **tsp turmeric**
- 1 **tsp cinnamon**
- 1 **tsp ground ginger**
  salt, to taste
- 1/2 **cup golden raisins, soaked in hot water for 20 minutes and drained**
- 1/4 **cup blanched almonds, slivered**

4. Place a small skillet over medium heat. Add almonds. Toast for 5–10 minutes or until they are just golden and they release their aroma. Stir almonds into rice, and keep covered until serving.

5. When chicken is finished, remove from oven. Cover with foil. Let stand for 10 minutes, then carve, drizzle with pan juices, and serve with rice.

Healthy Living Tradition

Whenever using fresh orange juice in a recipe, grate the zest and reserve it for garnish. Orange zest can lend intense orange flavor to this dish and others.

Exchanges/Choices	Calories		390	Sodium	240mg
1 1/2 Starch	Calories from Fat		115	**Total Carbohydrate**	40g
1 Fruit	**Total Fat**		13.0g	Dietary Fiber	2g
3 Lean Meat	Saturated Fat		2.5g	Sugars	14g
1 1/2 Fat	Trans Fat		0.0g	**Protein**	29g
	Cholesterol		75mg		

Serves 6
Serving Size: 1/3 cup rice +
3-oz piece chicken

Tarragon is a celebrated herb in southern France. It is most commonly paired with chicken and is used to flavor olive oils, vinegars, sauces, and egg and vegetable dishes. Its unique anise flavor is a traditional component of the French *fines herbes* trio of tarragon, parsley, and chervil.

Chicken Thighs with Tomato-Tarragon Sauce

1. Heat the olive oil in a large, wide skillet over medium heat. Add the chicken, and brown on all sides. Add vinegar, increase heat to high, and bring to a boil. Reduce heat to low, cover, and simmer for 10 minutes. Turn the chicken over, cover, and cook for another 10 minutes or until juices run clear from meat when pierced with a fork.

2. Remove chicken from pan. Add tomatoes and tarragon. Stir flour into sauce, and mix well to thicken. Season with salt and pepper. Return chicken to the pan. Increase heat to high. Bring to a boil, and reduce heat to low. Cover. Cook for 30 minutes. Serve warm.

2 Tbsp extra-virgin olive oil
6 skinless chicken thighs (about 2 lb)
1/4 cup apple cider vinegar
1 1/2 cups no-salt-added diced tomatoes
1/4 cup fresh tarragon, finely chopped
2 Tbsp unbleached, all-purpose flour
Salt, to taste
Freshly ground pepper, to taste

Healthy Living Tradition

Removing skin from the chicken before cooking it is a great way to avoid extra fat and calories. This way, the chicken is infused with flavor, and no one is tempted to eat the skin.

Exchanges/Choices			
1/2 Carbohydrate	Calories	220	Sodium	90mg
3 Lean Meat	Calories from Fat	115	Total Carbohydrate	5g
1 Fat	Total Fat	13.0g	Dietary Fiber	1g
	Saturated Fat	2.8g	Sugars	2g
	Trans Fat	0.0g	Protein	20g
Serves 6	Cholesterol	70mg		
Serving Size: 1 piece chicken			

This light, satisfying entrée contains the flavors of a classic chicken soup recipe. In Italy, mellow dishes like this are served during the winter months, while someone is getting over a cold, or whenever someone needs a break from spicy or complex dishes.

Chicken with Carrots and Leeks

1. Heat olive oil in a large, wide skillet. Season chicken with salt and pepper, and brown on all sides. Remove from pan.

2. Add carrots to pan. Brown on all sides. Add leeks. Season with salt and pepper. Return chicken to the pan. Cover with stock, and add coriander. Increase heat to high, and bring to a boil. Reduce heat to medium low, cover, and simmer for 20 minutes or until chicken is cooked through. Garnish with parsley. Serve hot.

2	**Tbsp extra-virgin olive oil**
1 1/2	**lb chicken breasts, sliced into 4-inch medallions**
	Salt, to taste
	Freshly ground pepper, to taste
4	**carrots, peeled and cut into 3-inch slices**
8	**leeks, rinsed well, trimmed to light green core, and diced**
1 1/2	**cups fat-free, low-sodium chicken stock**
2	**Tbsp coriander**
2	**Tbsp fresh parsley**

Healthy Living Tradition

Mediterranean lore is full of tales about leeks. Leeks belong to the allium family, which also contains onions and garlic. Try adding leeks to recipes in addition to onions and garlic for additional flavor and nutrients.

Exchanges/Choices			
4 Vegetable	**Calories**	350	
4 Lean Meat	Calories from Fat	100	
1 1/2 Fat	**Total Fat**	11.0g	
	Saturated Fat	2.2g	
	Trans Fat	0.0g	
Serves 4	**Cholesterol**	100mg	
Serving Size: 4 oz chicken + 1/2 cup vegetables			

Sodium	340mg
Total Carbohydrate	23g
Dietary Fiber	4g
Sugars	5g
Protein	39g

The word *fattah* comes from the Arabic word *fattat*, which means "well-grown girl." In this sense, the word refers to an ingredient that has been "grown" by adding other things to it, such as a casserole or panade. In Lebanon, where yogurt is a staple ingredient, shredded chicken is topped with chickpeas and yogurt spread. Another dish born of this tradition is the *Fattoush Salad* (p. 182).

Chicken Fattah

1. Combine drained yogurt and garlic, and set aside.

2. Place chicken in a large saucepan, and cover with water. Bring to a boil over high heat. Remove scum as it appears. Add onion, carrot, cinnamon stick, cardamom pods, cloves, peppercorns, and salt. Simmer, uncovered, for 30–45 minutes or until chicken is cooked through and tender. Remove chicken from pot. Strain the stock into another bowl or pot. Discard cinnamon. When chicken is cool enough to handle, shred it into large chunks.

3. Preheat oven to 350°F. Place pita pieces onto a baking sheet. Toast on each side until golden (about 3–4 minutes per side). Place pitas on the bottom of a baking dish. Ladle stock over the bread until it is soaked. Cover with chickpeas and chicken. Bake for 20 minutes or until thoroughly heated. Spoon yogurt-garlic mixture over the dish.

2	cups fat-free plain yogurt, drained in a fine sieve for at least 1 hour
2	cloves garlic, crushed
2	lb boneless, skinless chicken breasts
1	large onion, cut in half
1	large carrot, cut into pieces
1	cinnamon stick
5	green cardamom pods, crushed
5	whole cloves
5	peppercorns
1 1/4	tsp salt
3	pita breads, torn or cut into bite-size pieces
1	(14-oz) can chickpeas, drained
1	tsp extra-virgin olive oil
2/3	cup pine nuts

4. Heat olive oil in a small frying pan. Toast pine nuts until golden. Sprinkle pine nuts over the casserole and serve hot.

Healthy Living Tradition

Try adopting the Lebanese tradition of "growing" dishes by adding nutritious ingredients, such as beans and yogurt, to them.

Exchanges/Choices					
1 1/2 Starch	Calories	340	Sodium	545mg
4 Lean Meat	Calories from Fat	110	Total Carbohydrate	25g
1 Fat	Total Fat	12.0g	Dietary Fiber	3g
	Saturated Fat	1.5g	Sugars	5g
	Trans Fat	0.0g	Protein	33g
Serves 8	Cholesterol	70mg		
Serving Size: about 1 cup				

Serve this slightly sweet and sour dish with *Saffron Couscous (p. 76)* or *Saffron Rice with Almonds and Raisins* (p. 66). It tastes just as delicious the next day. If you are making this dish in advance, bring it to room temperature after cooking. Cover and refrigerate. The next day, reheat over medium heat until warmed through.

Chicken Breasts with Kumquats

1. Heat olive oil in a large, wide skillet over medium heat. Sprinkle chicken with *Moroccan Ras el Hanout Spice Mix*. Add to skillet. Brown for about 5–8 minutes per side. Transfer chicken to a plate.

2. Add onions to the skillet. Sauté until tender and golden, about 10 minutes. Add chicken, and pour stock over the top. Increase heat to high, and bring to a boil. Reduce heat to low, and add kumquats, apricots, and dates. Cover. Simmer for 15 minutes or until sauce is thickened, chicken is cooked through, and fruit is plumped. With a slotted spoon, transfer chicken and fruit to a serving platter. Stir the honey into the sauce, and pour over the top.

- **2 Tbsp extra-virgin olive oil**
- **2 lb boneless, skinless chicken breasts, cut into 6 pieces**
- **1 tsp Moroccan Ras el Hanout Spice Mix (p. 284)**
- **2 yellow onions, sliced**
- **2 cups fat-free, low-sodium vegetable stock**
- **6 oz kumquats, quartered lengthwise and seeded**
- **4 oz dried apricots, roughly chopped**
- **4 oz dried dates, pitted and roughly chopped**
- **1 Tbsp honey**

Healthy Living Tradition

Kumquats are native to China and have been grown in the U.S. since the mid 19th century. Kumquats are shaped like a grape tomato and have an orange color and grapefruit-like taste. They can be eaten whole, skin and all. For cooking, it is best to remove the seeds by slicing the kumquat. They make great additions to breads, stews, soups, and chicken recipes wherever a sweet and sour flavor combination is needed.

Exchanges/Choices				
2 Fruit	Calories	365	Sodium	210mg
1 Vegetable	Calories from Fat	80	Total Carbohydrate	39g
5 Lean Meat	Total Fat	9.0g	Dietary Fiber	6g
	Saturated Fat	1.7g	Sugars	30g
	Trans Fat	0.0g	Protein	34g
Serves 6	Cholesterol	90mg		
Serving Size: 1 cutlet + 1/6 of sauce				

Stuffing chicken breasts with healthful ingredients and poaching them makes this recipe tasty and unique. You will get rave reviews when serving this dish to others. Serve with *Potato-Artichoke Torte* (p. 152) and *Mozzarella, Tomato, and Chickpea Salad* (p. 190).

Stuffed Chicken Breasts with Cucumber Cream

❋ *Petti di Pollo al Cetriolo* ❋

3/4	cup fat-free plain yogurt, drained overnight
5	boneless, skinless chicken breast cutlets (about 1 1/4 lb total)
1	egg white
1/2	tsp salt, and more to taste
	Freshly ground pepper, to taste
4	cloves garlic
1/4	cup fresh dill
2	cucumbers
	Juice of 1 lemon
1	cup fat-free, low-sodium vegetable stock

1. Place a colander in a bowl. Add yogurt. Set in the refrigerator for 6 hours or overnight.

2. Chop a cutlet into four or five pieces, and place in a food processor fitted with a metal blade. Add the egg white to the food processor, along with 1/2 tsp salt and a few twists of freshly ground pepper. Add garlic and dill. Purée the mixture until it has a smooth, even consistency. Scoop the mixture into a small bowl. Cover, and refrigerate for 15 minutes.

3. Meanwhile, cover a work surface with wax paper. Place remaining four cutlets on wax paper. Cover with more wax paper. Use a meat tenderizer to lightly pound and slightly stretch out the meat. Remove and discard the wax paper from the top of the chicken.

4. When filling mixture has chilled for 15 minutes, remove it from the refrigerator, and divide it evenly among the chicken breasts, making vertical lines of purée down the length of each one. Roll up each chicken breast, covering the purée completely. Wrap each chicken breast roll in foil, being sure to seal the ends and sides, so that each bundle is waterproof.

5. Bring a large saucepan full of water to a boil. Place aluminum bundles in water, and reduce heat to medium. Boil, uncovered, for 20–30 minutes or until chicken is cooked through. When finished, use tongs to transfer rolls to a plate. Let stand until foil is cool enough to touch.

6. Meanwhile, cut the cucumbers in half vertically (lengthwise), and remove the seeds with the back of a spoon or paring knife. Dice 1 1/2 cucumbers. Slice the remaining 1/2 cucumber for garnish.

7. Bring a medium saucepan 3/4 full of water to boil over high heat. Reduce heat to medium, and add cucumbers and more salt, if desired. Cook cucumbers for 3 minutes or until slightly tender, yet still crunchy. Drain, and plunge into a bath of cold water and ice.

8. To make the sauce, combine lemon juice and broth in a medium saucepan. Bring to a boil over high heat. Boil for 5 minutes or until mixture is reduced by half. Stir in the yogurt, taste, and season with salt and pepper, if necessary. Stir the cooked cucumbers into the sauce.

9. Carefully remove foil from chicken, making sure not to leave any pieces on chicken. Slice chicken rolls on the diagonal into four slices each. Arrange slices on a serving platter, and top with sauce. Garnish with leftover cucumbers.

Healthy Living Tradition

Cucumbers are rich in potassium, a nutrient believed to improve muscle flexibility and improve elasticity of the skin.

Exchanges/Choices	Calories	210	Sodium	435mg
2 Vegetable	Calories from Fat	30	**Total Carbohydrate**	10g
4 Lean Meat	**Total Fat**	3.5g	Dietary Fiber	1g
	Saturated Fat	1.0g	Sugars	4g
Serves 4	Trans Fat	0.0g	**Protein**	34g
Serving Size: 1 chicken breast + 1/4 of sauce	**Cholesterol**	85mg		

These delicious, moist, and flavorful meatballs are sure to become a family favorite. You can also make larger 3- or 4-inch patties into healthy hamburgers using the same cooking method. To save time, double this recipe and use half of the meatballs to make the *Escarole and Meatball Soup* (p. 64).

Grandma's Chicken Meatballs

1. Grease a baking sheet with olive oil. Preheat the oven to 350°F. Pour 1/4 cup water onto the bottom of the baking sheet. Set aside.

2. Mix bread crumbs, chicken, onion, garlic, cilantro, coriander, 1/4 tsp salt, a few twists of freshly ground pepper, and mustard in a medium bowl. Roll the mixture into 1-inch balls. Place on the baking sheet.

3. Bake meatballs in the center of the oven for about 30 minutes or until cooked through.

1 tsp extra-virgin olive oil
1/2 cup plain, dry bread crumbs
1 lb ground chicken
1 medium yellow onion, finely chopped
3 cloves garlic, minced
1 bunch fresh cilantro, finely chopped
1 tsp ground coriander
1/4 tsp salt
   Freshly ground pepper, to taste
1 tsp Dijon mustard

Healthy Living Tradition

Adding flavorful ingredients like fresh cilantro, dried coriander, and onions to meatballs gives them so much flavor that no one will mind that they're baked instead of fried.

Exchanges/Choices		Calories	160	Sodium	230mg
1/2 Starch		Calories from Fat	65	**Total Carbohydrate**	10g
2 Lean Meat		**Total Fat**	7.0g	Dietary Fiber	1g
1/2 Fat		Saturated Fat	1.9g	Sugars	2g
		Trans Fat	0.0g	**Protein**	14g
Serves 6		**Cholesterol**	55mg		
Serving Size: 6 meatballs					

This delightful, nutritious dish is simple enough for daily meals, but special and delicious enough for festivities. Tarragon has a sweet anise flavor that marries well with the earthiness of the mushrooms. Feel free to use whatever mushrooms you like.

Tarragon Supreme of Chicken with Mushrooms

1. Heat olive oil in a large, wide skillet over medium heat. Add the garlic and tarragon, and sauté until garlic begins to release its aroma. Add lemon juice, lemon zest, stock, mushrooms, and pepper. Add the chicken, and sauté on each side until opaque and cooked through, about 10–15 minutes. Transfer chicken to a warm serving platter.

2. Increase heat to high. Cook for 3–5 minutes or until sauce is thickened and mushrooms are tender. Spoon sauce over chicken, and serve immediately.

2 Tbsp extra-virgin olive oil
2 Tbsp garlic, minced
2 Tbsp fresh tarragon, minced
1/4 cup freshly squeezed lemon juice
   Grated zest of 1 lemon
1/2 cup fat-free, low-sodium chicken stock
1 pint button mushrooms, scrubbed and trimmed
   Freshly ground pepper, to taste
4 boneless, skinless chicken breasts (about 2 lbs total), sliced in half and lightly pounded

Healthy Living Tradition

Double this recipe, and use leftover chicken to make sandwiches the next day.

Exchanges/Choices		Calories	165	Sodium	65mg
3 Lean Meat		Calories from Fat	55	**Total Carbohydrate**	2g
1/2 Fat		**Total Fat**	6.0g	Dietary Fiber	0g
		Saturated Fat	1.3g	Sugars	0g
Serves 8		Trans Fat	0.0g	**Protein**	25g
Serving Size: 1/2 chicken breast		**Cholesterol**	65mg		

This delicious date and chicken tajine evokes the tales of *One Thousand and One Nights* as its intoxicating spices waft in the air.

One Thousand and One Nights Chicken

1. Heat 2 Tbsp olive oil in a large skillet over medium-high heat. Sauté chicken pieces on each side until golden brown. Remove from pan, and set aside.

2. Add onion, cinnamon, cardamom, pepper, cumin, 1/2 tsp saffron, and chili powder to skillet. Stir, and sauté until onions are tender. Return chicken to skillet, and add cornstarch-and-stock mix and dates. Stir, and lower heat to medium low. Cover, and simmer for 45 minutes or until chicken is cooked through and dates are tender.

3. While chicken is simmering, bring 2 cups water and 1 tsp saffron to a boil, uncovered, in a medium saucepan with a lid. When water is boiling, remove pan from heat and add couscous. Mix well, cover pan with lid, and let stand for 5–10 minutes. Remove lid, and add remaining 1 Tbsp olive oil. Stir, add salt, and fluff with a fork. Spoon couscous onto a large serving platter.

3 **Tbsp extra-virgin olive oil, divided**
2 **lb boneless, skinless chicken breasts, sliced in half along the width**
1 **medium onion, diced**
1 **tsp ground cinnamon**
1 **tsp cardamom pods**
1/2 **tsp black pepper**
1 **tsp cumin**
1 1/2 **tsp saffron, divided**
1/2 **tsp chili powder**
2 **tsp cornstarch, dissolved in 2 cups fat-free, low-sodium chicken stock**
1/2 **lb dried dates, pitted**
2 **cups couscous**
Salt, to taste
Juice of 1 lemon
1/2 **cup roasted almonds, slivered**

4. Remove cardamom pods from chicken tajine. Arrange chicken on top of couscous. Squeeze lemon juice over the top. Sprinkle roasted almonds on top. Serve immediately.

Healthy Living Tradition

If you want to make this dish ahead of time, prepare the chicken tajine, allow it to cool completely, and store it in the refrigerator overnight. The next day, it can be reheated while the couscous is being prepared.

Exchanges/Choices					
3 Starch	Calories	615	Sodium	260mg
2 Fruit	Calories from Fat	145	**Total Carbohydrate**	76g
5 Lean Meat	**Total Fat**	16.0g	Dietary Fiber	7g
1 Fat	Saturated Fat	2.4g	Sugars	26g
	Trans Fat	0.0g	**Protein**	43g
	Cholesterol	90mg		

Serves 6
Serving Size: 1/2 cup couscous +
1/3 lb tajine

Cornish hens were first bred in the 20th century. Braising and roasting are the most popular methods of preparing them. This recipe is great for people who don't want to spend to much time in the kitchen, because once the hens go into the oven, you do not have any other "active" work to do.

Herb-Roasted Cornish Hens with Potatoes

1. Preheat oven to 425°F. Grease a 9 × 13-inch baking dish with 1 Tbsp olive oil. Place hens in dish. Place 1/2 lemon in the cavity of each one. Rub the skin of each hen with 1 Tbsp olive oil, and sprinkle each hen with 1/2 tsp *Herbes de Provence* and salt. Lay potato cubes around hens in dish. Cover with foil, and bake for 1–1 1/2 hours or until juices from the thigh joint run clear when pierced, basting every 30 minutes with pan juices. Remove from oven. Let stand, covered, for 10 minutes. Baste again, and serve warm.

5 **Tbsp extra-virgin olive oil, divided**
4 **Cornish hens (about 1 lb each), rinsed and dried**
2 **lemons, halved**
2 **tsp Herbes de Provence (p. 277)**
   Salt, to taste
1 **lb Yukon Gold potatoes, cubed**

Healthy Living Tradition

Roasts are perfect for busy schedules because you can put them in the oven and forget about them, using the time to do something else. Be sure to use any leftover meat to create Chicken Pita Sandwiches (p. 84) *or add it to your favorite soups and stews.*

Exchanges/Choices		Calories	215	Sodium	65mg
1/2 Starch		Calories from Fat	80	**Total Carbohydrate**	9g
3 Lean Meat		**Total Fat**	9.0g	Dietary Fiber	1g
1 Fat		Saturated Fat	1.6g	Sugars	0g
		Trans Fat	0.0g	**Protein**	23g
Serves 8		**Cholesterol**	100mg		
Serving Size: 1/2 Cornish hen + 1/2 cup roasted potatoes					

This dish has become the crown jewel of my American Thanksgiving meal. The combination of herbs, garlic, spices, and lemon juice create a flavorful, moist turkey that is simple to prepare. Turkey should be roasted 20–25 minutes per pound.

Southern French-Style Herb-Roasted Turkey

1. Preheat oven to 425°F. Use 1 Tbsp olive oil to grease the bottom of a large roasting pan. Wash and dry the turkey thoroughly. Season with salt and pepper on the inside and out. Place turkey breast side up in the pan. Brush the turkey with the remaining olive oil. Sprinkle *Herbes de Provence* and poultry seasoning on turkey, and rub into skin with your hands. Place whole garlic head, 1 lemon half, rosemary, thyme, and sage inside the cavity. Squeeze lemon juice from remaining lemon half over the top of the turkey. Place turkey in the oven, add a cup of water to the bottom of the pan, and roast for 1 hour, uncovered. Baste turkey after the first hour of cooking. If turkey looks very brown, cover it with foil. Continue to bake for another 2–2 1/2 hours or until the internal temperature of the thickest part of the turkey breast meat reads 180°F on a meat thermometer. Remove from the oven, and place on a carving board. Let rest for 10 minutes before carving. Remove skin while carving.

2. Strain the liquid from the bottom of the pan into another saucepan. Juice the remaining 2 lemon halves, add to the saucepan, and stir. Bring to a boil over high heat, and cook for 10 minutes or until sauce has reduced. Taste, and adjust seasoning if necessary. Serve sauce in a gravy boat next to turkey.

1/4 cup extra-virgin olive oil, divided
1 (10–12 lb) turkey
   Salt, to taste
   Freshly ground pepper, to taste
1 Tbsp Herbes de Provence (p. 277)
1 tsp poultry seasoning
1 whole head garlic, top chopped off
2 lemons, halved
1 sprig fresh rosemary
1 sprig fresh thyme
1 sprig fresh sage

Healthy Living Tradition

Much leaner than red meat, turkey doesn't need to be saved for Thanksgiving. Serve this delicious roast whenever you have a large gathering.

Exchanges/Choices		Calories	215	Sodium	80mg
4 Lean Meat		Calories from Fat	70	**Total Carbohydrate**	3g
1/2 Fat		**Total Fat**	8.0g	Dietary Fiber	2g
		Saturated Fat	2.2g	Sugars	0g
Serves 10		Trans Fat	0.0g	**Protein**	31g
Serving Size: 1/4 lb turkey meat		**Cholesterol**	80mg		

This recipe has replaced traditional beef hamburgers in my household. Packed with the bold flavors of dill and feta, this recipe is an updated classic. Try serving with recipe with the *Cucumber, String Bean, and Olive Tapenade Salad* (p. 186). The combination of fresh and cooked vegetables paired with fruity olive flavor of this salad make it a great alternative to French fries.

Dill and Feta Turkey Burgers

1. Preheat the oven to 425°F.

2. Combine turkey, mustard, dill, salt, and pepper in a large bowl. Stir to combine. Divide the meat into four equal portions, and form into patties.

3. Heat oil in a large oven-proof skillet over medium heat. Add burgers. Sauté for 2–3 minutes per side or until brown. Transfer to the oven, and cook for 15 minutes or until cooked through. Top with feta cheese, and cook for another 5 minutes or until cheese is melted. Serve on buns with a salad.

- 1 lb extra-lean ground turkey breast
- 1 Tbsp Dijon mustard
- 1/2 cup fresh dill, finely chopped
- 1/4 tsp kosher salt
  Freshly ground pepper, to taste
- 1 Tbsp extra virgin olive oil
- 2 oz crumbled low-fat feta cheese
- 4 (2-oz) fresh bakery whole-wheat buns

Healthy Living Tradition

These burgers freeze well. Why not make a double batch, and freeze half for later?

Exchanges/Choices	Calories	335	Sodium	710mg
2 Starch	Calories from Fat	80	**Total Carbohydrate**	30g
4 Lean Meat	**Total Fat**	9.0g	Dietary Fiber	4g
	Saturated Fat	2.4g	Sugars	6g
Serves 4	Trans Fat	0.0g	**Protein**	36g
Serving Size: 1 burger	**Cholesterol**	60mg		

Thin slices of quick-cooking veal cutlets like these are the go-to dishes for busy working women in the Mediterranean. Veal can be cooked in minutes, yet still offers luxurious, succulent flavors that the whole family loves. The smoky roasted red peppers deepen the complexity of the dish, which is offset by the fresh, peppery flavor of arugula. Serve with *Corn, Tomato, Pea, and Dill Salad* (p. 185) for an unbelievable flavor and color. It's best to call your local supermarket or butcher to make sure they have veal on hand before making this recipe.

Veal Scaloppine with Roasted Red Peppers and Arugula

1. Place flour on a large plate. Season with salt and pepper, stirring to combine. Dip veal pieces into flour, and turn to coat, shake off excess, and place on a platter.

2. Heat 2 Tbsp oil in a large, wide nonstick oven-proof skillet.

3. Preheat oven broiler.

4. Add veal to skillet, and cook for 2–3 minutes per side, turning only once, until meat is cooked through.

5. Toss arugula with remaining 2 Tbsp extra-virgin olive oil.

1/2 cup unbleached, all-purpose flour
1/4 tsp kosher salt
    Freshly ground pepper, to taste
6 pieces (about 1/4 lb each) veal scaloppine
4 Tbsp extra-virgin olive oil, divided
5 oz baby arugula
4 jarred roasted red peppers, drained well
1/4 cup balsamic vinegar

6. Place roasted red peppers in a food processor. Process for a few seconds, until a purée is formed.

7. To serve, divide arugula among six plates. Place veal slice next to arugula. Top each slice with pepper purée. Drizzle balsamic vinegar over the top of each plate. Top with a twist of freshly ground pepper.

Healthy Living Tradition

Lately, a lot of cooking shows on television talk about "developing a relationship" with butchers and fishmongers. This concept is completely foreign to most Americans because we can walk into stores and find most of what we need right there. I enjoy getting to know the people who grow, produce, and sell my food for a number of reasons. When dealing with butchers in particular, you can learn a lot and save time by getting to know them. Veal scaloppine, for example, is something that is tricky and time consuming to cut at home. A butcher will be able to cut perfectly thin slices for you. He or she can also make sure that each piece weighs exactly what you need for portion control. Butchers and fishmongers can also order special cuts of meat, advise you on which meats are the freshest, and let you know about special values.

Exchanges/Choices		Calories	255	Sodium	150mg
1/2 Carbohydrate		Calories from Fat	115	Total Carbohydrate	10g
4 Lean Meat		Total Fat	13.0g	Dietary Fiber	1g
1 Fat		Saturated Fat	2.3g	Sugars	3g
		Trans Fat	0.0g	Protein	26g
Serves 6		Cholesterol	75mg		
Serving Size: 1 piece veal					

This is a wonderful roast to make in the fall and winter. Traditionally, roasts were made during the cooler periods in the Mediterranean because the oven played a key role in warming the home. Here, the vegetables are puréed to make a sauce that is poured over the sliced roast. If you prefer to serve the vegetables whole, add them to the pan during the last hour of cooking, so they will not be overdone.

Roasted Veal with Root Vegetables

1. Preheat oven to 400°F. Heat olive oil in an oven-proof casserole or pan over medium-high heat. Add veal roast, and brown on all sides. Add carrots, celery, onion, sweet potatoes, parsnips, garlic, salt, and pepper. Stir. Bring to a boil over high heat. Squeeze lime juice over the roast. Add coriander, cinnamon stick, chicken stock, and tomatoes to the pan. Stir, remove from heat, and cover. Place roast in the oven, and cook for 2 hours or until veal is tender.

2. Place veal on a cutting board. Let rest for 10 minutes. Remove cinnamon stick, and discard.

3. While the roast is resting, transfer half of the sauce and vegetables to a blender. Remove the center spout of the lid, and cover with a kitchen towel. Purée into a smooth sauce. Taste, and adjust salt if necessary.

4. Slice veal. Arrange vegetables around it on a serving platter. Pour sauce over the top, and serve warm.

2 Tbsp extra-virgin olive oil
1 (3 lb) boneless breast of veal roast, trimmed of fat
1/2 lb carrots (about 3), chopped
1/2 lb celery stalks (about 3), chopped
1/2 cup chopped yellow onion (about 1)
1 lb sweet potatoes (about 3), chopped
1/2 lb parsnips (about 2), peeled and chopped
2 cloves garlic, chopped
1 tsp salt
1/2 tsp freshly ground pepper
Juice of 1 lime (about 2 Tbsp)
1 tsp coriander
1 cinnamon stick
2 cups fat-free, low-sodium chicken stock
1 cup chopped or diced no-salt-added tomatoes

Healthy Living Tradition

Making roasts on the weekend is a Mediterranean tradition. Roasts taste great and require little effort to make. Although they can feed large crowds, they are still worth making for one or two. You can eat them as a traditional meal; use leftovers in salads, sandwiches, and pasta dishes; and freeze the rest for later.

Exchanges/Choices			Calories	200	Sodium	295mg
1/2 Starch • 1 Vegetable			Calories from Fat	70	**Total Carbohydrate**	12g
2 Lean Meat • 1 Fat			**Total Fat**	8.0g	Dietary Fiber	2g
			Saturated Fat	2.6g	Sugars	4g
Serves 12			Trans Fat	0.0g	**Protein**	20g
Serving Size: 3 oz veal + 1/2 cup vegetables/sauce			**Cholesterol**	70mg		

One of my favorite dishes is Sultan's Delight, a Turkish dish invented for Sultan Murad IV, which consists of slowly simmered lamb morsels served over an eggplant-béchamel sauce. I created this dish as a quick version that offers some of the same flavors any time. *Chickpeas and Rice* (p. 67) is a great accompaniment to this dish.

Veal Scaloppine with Eggplant Veloutè

1. Preheat broiler.

2. Place yogurt in a fine sieve or strainer over a bowl to drain. Pierce eggplants with a fork, and place on a baking sheet under broiler. Broil for 10–15 minutes, turning once, until blackened and blistered. Set eggplants aside in a colander to drain.

3. Heat olive oil over medium heat in a large, wide skillet. Pat scaloppine dry, and season with salt and pepper. Add to skillet, and cook for 2–3 minutes per side, until browned. Add tomato purée and stock. Bring to a boil. Reduce heat to low, cover, and simmer for 5–10 minutes.

1/2	cup low-fat, plain yogurt
2	large eggplants
1	Tbsp extra-virgin olive oil
2	lb veal scaloppine, sliced into 6 slices
	Kosher salt, to taste
	Freshly ground pepper, to taste
1	cup tomato purée (no added salt or fat)
1	cup fat-free, low-sodium chicken stock

4. When eggplants are cool enough to touch, peel them and place them back in the colander over the sink or a bowl. Mash the eggplants with a potato masher, and transfer the eggplant pulp to a saucepan over medium heat. Season eggplant with salt and pepper to taste. When eggplant is warm, remove from heat, and stir in yogurt, mixing well to incorporate.

5. Spread eggplant onto the bottom of a serving dish. Remove veal pieces from the pan with tongs. Place them on top of eggplant. Increase the heat under the veal sauce skillet to high, and cook for a few minutes to thicken, stirring the bottom with a wooden spoon to dislodge any bits of meat. Strain the sauce over the veal, and serve immediately.

Healthy Living Tradition

Eggplants are a great source of soluble fiber and are low in carbohydrate.

Exchanges/Choices		Calories	255	Sodium	175mg
2 Vegetable		Calories from Fat	65	**Total Carbohydrate**	11g
4 Lean Meat		**Total Fat**	7.0g	Dietary Fiber	3g
1/2 Fat		Saturated Fat	1.9g	Sugars	5g
		Trans Fat	0.0g	**Protein**	35g
Serves 6		**Cholesterol**	105mg		
Serving Size: 1 piece of veal + 1/6 eggplant veloute					

Psari plaki **means "baked fish" in Greek.** This recipe is a traditional Greek-style fish that is baked with many savory ingredients, making it a perfect meal in one. Popular throughout Greece, this dish is made from a wide variety of fish, including salted cod, sea bass, mullet, halibut, and red snapper. For convenience, fish fillets can be substituted. A common addition, which I have left out of this version, is raisins, which give a sweet and sour flavor to the fish. Serve this dish with a small piece of feta cheese, olives, crusty bread, and a tossed salad with extra-virgin olive oil and lemon juice.

Greek-Style Baked Fish ❋ Psari Plaki ❋

1. Preheat oven to 350°F. Grease the bottom of an 11 × 17-inch baking dish with 1 tsp olive oil. Place parsley, potatoes, spinach, pepper slices, diced tomato, garlic, and oregano on the bottom of the pan, layering each one on top of the other. Season the fish with salt and pepper, and lay on top of vegetable mixture.

2. Add 1/4 cup olive oil, flour, and paprika to a small bowl or measuring cup, and whisk vigorously to incorporate with a fork. Pour the mixture over the fish. Pour 1/2 cup water over all the herbs and vegetables on the sides of the pan. Place tomato slices on top of the fish. Season with sea salt and ground pepper to taste. Bake 40–45 minutes or until fish is opaque and flakes easily when pierced with a fork. Carefully remove the fish from the baking dish, and serve each plate with a bed of vegetables on the bottom, a fish fillet on the top, and spoon sauce over the top and sides to finish.

- 1/4 cup + 1 tsp extra-virgin olive oil, divided
- 1 bunch fresh parsley, chopped
- 1 1/2 lb (about 4 medium Yukon Gold) potatoes, cut into very thin slices
- 2 (10-oz) pkgs frozen spinach, thawed and drained well
- 2 Cubanelle peppers, sliced into rings
- 2 medium tomatoes, 1 diced and 1 halved and cut into slices
- 5 cloves garlic, roughly chopped
- 4 Tbsp fresh oregano, finely chopped, or 1 Tbsp dried
- 6 (1/3 lb each) cod, red snapper, sea bass, or halibut fillets
  Sea salt, to taste
  Freshly ground pepper, to taste
- 2 Tbsp unbleached, all-purpose flour
- 1 tsp sweet paprika

Healthy Living Tradition

It's great to have a repertoire of healthful, easy, one-dish recipes that can be made on busy weeknights. Keep canned tomatoes and frozen fish and vegetables on hand for when fresh ones aren't in season.

Exchanges/Choices					
1 1/2 Starch	Calories	385	Sodium	180mg
2 Vegetable	Calories from Fat	110	**Total Carbohydrate**	39g
4 Lean Meat	**Total Fat**	12.0g	Dietary Fiber	7g
1 Fat	Saturated Fat	1.6g	Sugars	3g
	Trans Fat	0.0g	**Protein**	34g
	Cholesterol	65mg		

Serves 6
Serving Size: 1/6 recipe

This dish is a classic Middle Eastern treat. The creamy texture and nutty, citrusy taste of tahini sauce perfectly complements the mild-flavored white fish.

Fish with Tahini Sauce

1. Rinse tilapia fillets and pat dry.

2. Combine salt, pepper, *Seafood Seasoning*, and flour in a shallow bowl.

3. Heat olive oil in a large, wide skillet over medium-high heat. Dredge fish fillets in flour. Dust off excess. Place fillets in pan, and brown for 3–5 minutes per side or until cooked through. Serve with *Tahini Sauce* and lemon wedges, with steamed cauliflower on the side.

4	tilapia fillets (each about 4 oz)
1/2	tsp sea salt
1/4	tsp freshly ground black pepper
2	Tbsp Seafood Seasoning (p. 287)
1/4	cup flour
1 3/4	Tbsp extra-virgin olive oil
1	lemon, thinly sliced
1/2	recipe Tahini Sauce (p. 279)
4	lemon wedges
4	cups steamed cauliflower

Healthy Living Tradition

Pan-frying is a healthier alternative to deep-frying. In the Mediterranean, poultry, fish, meat, and vegetables are often cooked this way. Full-bodied seasoning combinations are used to compensate for the deep-fried flavor in pan-fried dishes.

Exchanges/Choices				
1/2 Starch	Calories	275	Sodium	425mg
1 Vegetable	Calories from Fat	115	**Total Carbohydrate**	14g
1 Lean Meat	**Total Fat**	13.0g	Dietary Fiber	5g
1 1/2 Fat	Saturated Fat	2.4g	Sugars	3g
	Trans Fat	0.0g	**Protein**	27g
	Cholesterol	75mg		

Serves 4
Serving Size: 1 fish fillet

Chermoula sauce is a Moroccan classic that tastes great on both chicken and fish. This recipe is prepared in the style of Eoussaria, a coastal Moroccan town where seafood is an integral part of daily life. There, locals and tourists buy fresh fish directly from fishermen. They then bring the fish to a road-side restaurant or stand to be cleaned, dressed, and prepared to their specifications. While this recipe calls for fish steaks, fish is generally roasted whole in Morocco.

Fish with Chermoula Sauce

❈ Samak bi Chermoula ❈

1. Preheat oven to 425°F. Grease a large baking dish with 1 Tbsp olive oil. Place fish skin side down in the bottom of the dish, and make a few slash marks on top of each piece.

2. Mix together the cilantro, parsley, garlic, salt, paprika, and lemon juice. Stir in remaining olive oil. Spread half of the sauce over the fish, and rub it into the slash marks. Place potato, tomato, and pepper slices over fish. Top with remaining sauce. Cover with foil, and bake 20 minutes or until vegetables are tender and fish flakes easily. Sprinkle with lemon zest and serve.

- 3 Tbsp extra-virgin olive oil, divided
- 4 halibut, cod, or grouper steaks (4–5 oz each)
- 2 Tbsp finely chopped cilantro
- 2 Tbsp finely chopped parsley
- 6 cloves garlic, minced
- 3/4 tsp fine sea salt
- 1 tsp paprika
- 2 lemons, juiced and zested
- 1 large boiling potato, peeled and very thinly sliced
- 2 Roma tomatoes, thinly sliced
- 2 jalapeño pepper, if desired, sliced into rings

Healthy Living Tradition

Find ways to incorporate fresh fish into your diet, and experiment with different ways of preparing them. Seek out fishmongers and organic supermarkets that sell top-quality fish.

Exchanges/Choices	Calories	270	Sodium	515mg
1/2 Starch	Calories from Fat	115	**Total Carbohydrate**	14g
1 Vegetable	**Total Fat**	13.0g	Dietary Fiber	2g
3 Lean Meat	Saturated Fat	1.8g	Sugars	2g
1 1/2 Fat	Trans Fat	0.0g	**Protein**	25g
	Cholesterol	35mg		

Serves 4
Serving Size: 1 piece fish

Warm homemade couscous dished up with ladles of fresh seafood in spiced broth is a Tunisian specialty. This North African dish is the crowning glory of elaborate holiday buffets. Each family has its own recipe. Depending on the season, and individual tastes, the couscous may contain chickpeas, potatoes, numerous spices, mussels, prawns, cream, and hot sauces. This is a simple version that is perfect for special occasions and weeknight indulgences. Serve with *Moroccan Harissa Sauce* (p. 278) and *Tomato and Pepper Salad* (p. 179).

Tunisian Fish Couscous

❋ *CusCus bil Samak* ❋

1. Bring 2 cups fish stock, onion, cumin, saffron, chili powder, salt, and pepper to a boil in a medium saucepan over high heat. Add fish, reduce heat to low, stir gently, cover, and simmer for 10 minutes or until fish is opaque and cooked through.

2. Meanwhile, bring remaining 1 1/2 cups fish stock to a boil in a medium saucepan over high heat. Remove stock from the heat. Add the couscous, stir, and cover. Let stand for 10 minutes. Remove lid, fluff couscous, and pour onto a serving platter. Ladle fish and stock on top of the couscous and serve hot.

3 1/2 **cups reduced-sodium fish stock, divided**
1 **large yellow onion, thinly sliced**
1 **tsp cumin**
1/2 **tsp saffron**
Pinch chili powder
1/2 **tsp unrefined sea salt, divided**
1/4 **tsp black pepper**
2 1/2 **lb fresh fish fillets (such as bass or cod)**
2 **cups couscous**

Healthy Living Tradition

In addition to the many nutritional advantages to its credit, some fish is also naturally low in saturated fats.

Exchanges/Choices		Calories	435	Sodium	545mg
3 Starch		Calories from Fat	45	Total Carbohydrate	48g
5 Lean Meat		Total Fat	5.0g	Dietary Fiber	3g
		Saturated Fat	0.3g	Sugars	3g
Serves 6		Trans Fat	0.0g	Protein	46g
Serving Size: about 1 cup		Cholesterol	80mg		

This quintessential Roman recipe is both festive and delicious. Let this dish be the main course of a classic Italian meal by serving it with *Roman Spaghetti with Artichokes, Mint, and Garlic* (p. 74), *Romaine, Spinach, and Radicchio Salad* (p. 172), and *Fresh Figs with Raspberry Purée* (p. 229). Invite your friends and family over to enjoy this feast.

Roasted Cod with Tomatoes, Zucchini, and Olives

1. Preheat oven to 425°F.

2. Place tomatoes, zucchini, and onion in a large baking dish, and season with salt and pepper. Drizzle with olive oil, and roast for about 20 minutes or until vegetables are tender.

3. Remove from oven, and stir in garlic, olives, and basil. Place cod fillets on top of vegetables, and sprinkle with salt and pepper. Drizzle with lime juice. Return to oven. Bake for about 15 minutes, until fish is cooked through.

1 cup Roma tomatoes, diced
2 large zucchini, diced
1 yellow onion, sliced
Salt, to taste
Freshly ground black pepper, to taste
2 Tbsp extra-virgin olive oil
2 cloves garlic, chopped
1/4 cup kalamata olives, pitted and diced
1/4 cup basil, chopped
4 cod fillets (4–6 oz each)
Juice of 1 lime

Healthy Living Tradition

Cod is a mild-tasting staple fish used in most parts of the Mediterranean. Because fresh fish freezes well, you can buy the cod when it is on sale and store it in the freezer wrapped in freezer bags for up to 6 months.

Exchanges/Choices	Calories	215	Sodium	155mg
2 Vegetable	Calories from Fat	80	Total Carbohydrate	12g
3 Lean Meat	Total Fat	9.0g	Dietary Fiber	3g
1/2 Fat	Saturated Fat	1.3g	Sugars	6g
	Trans Fat	0.0g	Protein	23g
Serves 4	Cholesterol	50mg		

Serving Size: 1 cod fillet + 1/2 cup of vegetables

When directly translated to English, the Italian name for this dish is "fish in crazy water." The "crazy" refers to the addition of crushed red pepper flakes to an otherwise mild sauce. This recipe hails from the beautiful Amalfi coast. Any firm white fish can be substituted for the sea bass.

Poached Sea Bass with Tomatoes and Herbs

❋ Pesce all'acqua pazza ❋

1. Heat olive oil in a large, wide skillet over medium-high heat. Add garlic, celery, pepper flakes, and rosemary. Cook for 2 minutes. Add parsley, tomatoes, 1 cup water, and salt. Stir well to incorporate. Allow mixture to come to a boil. Carefully lower the fish fillets into the water. Season with pepper to taste. Reduce heat to low, and poach fish for 10–15 minutes or until it is cooked through. Be careful to keep the temperature below the boiling point, so the fish doesn't flake. Serve fish fillets in individual bowls with broth ladled over them.

2 Tbsp extra-virgin olive oil
2 cloves garlic, minced
1 celery stalk, minced
1/4 tsp crushed red pepper flakes
1 tsp fresh rosemary, finely chopped
1/4 cup fresh Italian parsley, finely chopped
1/2 lb cherry tomatoes, chopped
3/4 tsp fine sea salt
4 sea bass fillets (4–5 oz each)
Freshly ground pepper

Healthy Living Tradition

Poaching poultry and seafood is an easy and healthy alternative to frying. Try using the same method with other sources of protein.

Exchanges/Choices		Calories	185	Sodium	540mg
3 Lean Meat		Calories from Fat	80	Total Carbohydrate	3g
1 Fat		Total Fat	9.0g	Dietary Fiber	1g
		Saturated Fat	0.9g	Sugars	2g
Serves 4		Trans Fat	0.0g	Protein	22g
Serving Size: 1 piece fish		Cholesterol	45mg		

Fresh tuna and swordfish are plentiful around the shores of Sicily. This recipe combines many of Sicily's delicacies: olive oil, citrus fruits, capers, anchovies, and mint. This dish will impress guests, but can also be made on the busiest weeknights. Serve it with *Sicilian Salad with Potatoes* (p. 184) and Sicilian olives for an authentic weeknight meal.

Sicilian-Style Tuna Steaks

❀ *Tonno alla Siciliana* ❀

1. Heat olive oil in a large skillet over medium-high heat. Add tuna steaks. Cook 2–3 minutes per side until golden. Remove tuna from pan, and place on a platter. Set aside.

2. Add onion, capers, and anchovies to pan. Stir, and break up the anchovies with a wooden spoon. Sauté, uncovered, over medium heat, until onions are translucent (5–7 minutes). Add orange juice, stir well to combine, and cook, uncovered, for 2–3 minutes. Return tuna steaks to pan, cover, and cook for 3–5 minutes per side until tuna is done.*

3. Remove tuna from pan, and place on a serving platter. Pour sauce over tuna, and arrange onions around the top and sides of the platter. Season tuna with salt and pepper. Sprinkle mint on top of the dish. Serve warm.

2	**Tbsp extra-virgin olive oil**
4	**tuna steaks (4 oz each)**
1	**medium yellow onion, thinly sliced**
1	**Tbsp capers, packed in water, drained and rinsed well**
8	**anchovy fillets in olive oil, drained and rinsed well**
1/2	**cup freshly squeezed orange juice (1–2 oranges)**
1/4	**tsp salt**
	Freshly ground pepper, to taste
2	**Tbsp freshly chopped mint**

*Sicilians generally serve their tuna cooked through. If you like yours red in the middle, do not allow the tuna to cook for the full 5 minutes on each side.

Healthy Living Tradition

Serve these tuna steaks on whole-wheat buns and serve them for lunch as an elegant, healthy alternative to hamburgers or tuna salad sandwiches.

Exchanges/Choices	Calories	265	Sodium	545mg
1/2 Carbohydrate	Calories from Fat	115	**Total Carbohydrate**	7g
4 Lean Meat	**Total Fat**	13.0g	Dietary Fiber	1g
1 Fat	Saturated Fat	2.5g	Sugars	5g
	Trans Fat	0.0g	**Protein**	28g
	Cholesterol	50mg		
Serves 4				
Serving Size: 1 (4-oz) tuna steak				

Grilled fish is both healthy and flavorful. Cod, haddock, or turbot can also be used with this easy recipe.

Grilled Grouper with Moroccan Dipping Sauce

1. Combine coriander, cumin, pepper, paprika, lemon juice, lemon zest, garlic, olive oil, and yogurt in a medium bowl. Whisk to form a dressing. Pour half of the dressing into another bowl, and refrigerate it.

2. Place fish in a shallow dish. Pour the remaining dressing over the fish. Cover, and refrigerate for 1 hour. About 10 minutes before fish has finished marinating, preheat grill, grill pan, or broiler.

3. Grill or broil fish for about 5 minutes per side or until lightly golden and cooked through. (Fish should flake away in large chunks when it is fully cooked.) Season with salt. Serve immediately with dipping sauce on the side.

- 1 tsp ground coriander
- 1 tsp ground cumin
- 1/4 tsp freshly ground black pepper
- 1 tsp paprika
- 1/4 cup freshly squeezed lemon juice
  Zest of l lemon
- 1 clove garlic, minced
- 2 Tbsp extra-virgin olive oil
- 2 Tbsp fat-free Greek yogurt
- 4 boneless grouper fillets (4–5 oz each)
- 1/2 tsp salt

Healthy Living Tradition

Full of probiotics-friendly bacteria that help keep your gut in shape, yogurt is a wonderfully nutritious food on the market today. Make sure to choose a brand with active yogurt cultures. Try substituting it for mayonnaise and oil in your favorite dressing, marinade, and dip recipes.

Exchanges/Choices				
3 Lean Meat	Calories	160	Sodium	345mg
1/2 Fat	Calories from Fat	55	Total Carbohydrate	2g
	Total Fat	6.0g	Dietary Fiber	0g
	Saturated Fat	1.0g	Sugars	1g
Serves 4	Trans Fat	0.0g	Protein	23g
Serving Size: 1 fish fillet +	Cholesterol	40mg		
2 Tbsp sauce				

This is a simple, elegant way of serving salmon. Cabbage is a low-calorie wrapper for the salmon, enabling it to stay moist and juicy during cooking. Serve this dish with *Rice and Herb Stuffed Tomatoes* (p. 68).

Salmon-Stuffed Cabbage Leaves

1. Bring a large pot of water to boil over high heat. Clean cabbage by removing outer leaves and discarding them. Carefully peel off whole cabbage leaves. Place in boiling water. Boil cabbage until tender (about 10 minutes). Drain, and place in a bowl of ice water to cool. Drain again, remove the 8 largest leaves, and place them on a work surface.

2. Place salmon pieces on top of cabbage leaves. Season with salt and pepper. Roll sides of cabbage in, and roll up the salmon. Grease an oven-proof baking dish with olive oil. Place rolls seam side down in dish. Cut up remaining cabbage into bite-size pieces. Scatter around the dish. Pour vegetable stock over cabbage, and bake for 20 minutes or until salmon is cooked through. Serve salmon rolls on top of the excess cabbage while still hot.

1 **head cabbage (about 2 1/2 lb)**
1 **lb salmon, skin removed, cut into 8 equal pieces**
 Salt, to taste
 Freshly ground pepper, to taste
1 **Tbsp extra-virgin olive oil**
1 **cup fat-free, low-sodium vegetable stock**

Healthy Living Tradition

Protein-packed salmon is a great choice for people with diabetes because it is full of healthy omega-3 vitamins, which help lower cholesterol. Try to make salmon or other fatty fish a part of your weekly diet.

Exchanges/Choices	Calories	285	Sodium	115mg
3 Vegetable	Calories from Fat	125	Total Carbohydrate	13g
3 Lean Meat	Total Fat	14.0g	Dietary Fiber	4g
1 1/2 Fat	Saturated Fat	2.2g	Sugars	6g
	Trans Fat	0.0g	Protein	28g
Serves 4	Cholesterol	80mg		
Serving Size: 2 rolls + 1/2 cup cabbage				

Pink salmon is doled out on a gorgeous green bed of pea purée in this elegant dish, which I have seen served in Italy. If you are preparing this dish for a party, you can make the fish and the pea purée a day ahead of time and reheat them before serving. The citrusy flavors of the *Arborio Rice Salad and Vegetables* (p. 65) complement this dish well.

Salmon with Pea Purée

1. Combine peas, juice of 1 lemon, vegetable stock, salt, and pepper in a blender. Purée until smooth.

2. Preheat oven to 425°F. Grease a baking dish with olive oil. Place salmon in dish, and turn to coat with oil. Sprinkle each piece with *Seafood Seasoning* and juice of 1 lemon. Bake for 15–20 minutes or until salmon is cooked through.

3. Pour purée on the bottom of a serving platter. Place salmon on top. Garnish with lemon wedges.

1 **lb fresh sweet peas**
Juice of 2 lemons, divided
1/2 **cup fat-free, low-sodium vegetable stock**
1/4 **tsp salt**
Freshly ground black pepper, to taste
1 **tsp extra-virgin olive oil**
1 **lb salmon fillet, cut into 4 equal parts**
1 **tsp Seafood Seasoning (p. 287)**
1 **lemon, quartered**

Healthy Living Tradition

It's important to know how to choose fresh salmon fillets in order to get the best flavor from your dishes. When buying salmon fillets, look for firm-fleshed pieces that bounce back when pressed. The fillets should be moist with no discoloration. Fresh fish should smell like the ocean.

Exchanges/Choices	Calories	265	Sodium	395mg
1 Starch	Calories from Fat	100	**Total Carbohydrate**	11g
3 Lean Meat	**Total Fat**	11.0g	Dietary Fiber	3g
1 Fat	Saturated Fat	1.9g	Sugars	4g
	Trans Fat	0.0g	**Protein**	28g
Serves 4	**Cholesterol**	80mg		
Serving Size: 1 piece salmon				

This delicious main course is quick and easy to make. You can make the salmon rolls in the morning, keep them refrigerated, and cook them just before serving.

Salmon Stuffed with Spinach and Feta

1. Preheat oven to 350°F. Heat 1 Tbsp olive oil in skillet over medium heat. Add spinach, and stir to coat. Add feta, salt, pepper, and mint. Stir to combine, and remove from heat.

2. Grease bottom of a baking dish with remaining 1 Tbsp oil.

3. Place fillets on a work surface, and cover with 1/2 cup spinach mixture on each. Roll fillets up, and stand on one end. Place in baking dish, and turn to coat in olive oil. Season with salt and pepper. Pour stock into the bottom of the baking dish. Pour lemon juice on the top of the fillets. Cover with foil. Bake for 20 minutes or until salmon is cooked through.

- 2 **Tbsp extra-virgin olive oil, divided**
- 1 **(16-oz) bag frozen spinach, thawed and drained well**
- 2 **Tbsp reduced-fat feta cheese, crumbled**
  Salt, to taste
  Pepper, to taste
- 1 **tsp dried mint**
- 4 **salmon fillets (3.5 oz each), skinned**
- 2 **cups fat-free, low-sodium vegetable stock**
  Juice of 1 lemon

Healthy Living Tradition

We experience food through our senses of smell and sight long before we actually taste it. Attractive visual presentations, like the combination of green spinach and pink salmon, create a positive dining experience before we even start eating.

Exchanges/Choices					
1 Vegetable	**Calories**	285	**Sodium**	275mg
3 Lean Meat	Calories from Fat	155	**Total Carbohydrate**	7g
2 1/2 Fat	**Total Fat**	17.0g	Dietary Fiber	4g
	Saturated Fat	2.9g	Sugars	1g
	Trans Fat	0.0g	**Protein**	27g
Serves 4	**Cholesterol**	70mg		
Serving Size: 1 salmon roll				

Because swordfish is not always stocked in American supermarkets, it's a good idea to call ahead and find out when a shipment will be arriving and place an order. Pumpkin swordfish, tuna, haddock, and cod can all be substituted for white swordfish. Serve this dish with the *Potato-Artichoke Torte* (p. 152) and *Romaine, Spinach, and Radicchio Salad* (p. 172) for a fast and fabulous meal.

Swordfish with Tomatoes

1. Heat olive oil in a large skillet over medium heat. Add garlic, and cook until it releases its aroma. Do not let garlic turn brown. Stir in chopped and strained tomatoes, basil, 1/4 tsp salt, pepper, and pepper flakes. Stir and cover. Reduce heat to low, and simmer for 5 minutes. Slowly remove lid from tomato sauce, and add swordfish to simmering sauce.

2. Cover, and cook for 10–15 minutes or until fish is cooked through. Transfer fish to a serving platter. Top with remaining sauce. Season with remaining 1/4 tsp salt, if needed.

- **1 Tbsp extra-virgin olive oil**
- **2 cloves garlic, minced**
- **2 cups chopped boxed tomatoes or reduced-sodium canned diced tomatoes**
- **2 Tbsp freshly chopped basil**
- **1/2 tsp sea salt, divided**
- **1/8 tsp freshly grated pepper**
  Dash crushed red pepper flakes
- **4 boneless swordfish fillets (1/3 lb each)**

Healthy Living Tradition

In the Mediterranean region, high-quality wild fish is consumed on a regular basis and is believed to have an anti-inflammatory effect on the body.

Exchanges/Choices	Calories	240	Sodium	480mg
1 Vegetable	Calories from Fat	90	**Total Carbohydrate**	7g
4 Lean Meat	**Total Fat**	10.0g	Dietary Fiber	2g
1/2 Fat	Saturated Fat	2.1g	Sugars	4g
	Trans Fat	0.0g	**Protein**	31g
Serves 4	**Cholesterol**	60mg		
Serving Size: 1 fillet				

Swordfish and eggplant are culinary ingredients that Sicilians inherited when they were under Arab rule. Before the arrival of the Arabs, swordfish was not eaten because of its reputation as being extremely difficult to catch. Sicilian fisherman learned how to catch swordfish from the Arabs. Even today, Sicilian fisherman use Arabic words instead of Italian ones when fishing. Serve this delightful dish with *Baby Artichokes with Herb Sauce* (p. 150).

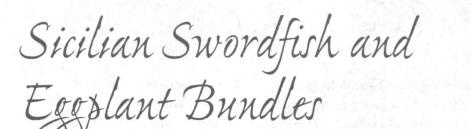

Sicilian Swordfish and Eggplant Bundles
❋ *Involtini di Pesce Spade e Melanzane* ❋

1. Preheat broiler. Place eggplant slices on a baking sheet. Brush with 1 Tbsp olive oil, and bake for a few minutes until tender and cooked through. Remove from oven, and set aside.

2. Heat remaining 1 Tbsp olive oil in a large skillet over medium heat. Add garlic, and cook until it releases its aroma. Do not let garlic turn brown. Stir in chopped and strained tomatoes, basil, pine nuts, 1/4 tsp salt, pepper, and pepper flakes. Stir and cover. Reduce heat to low. Simmer for 5 minutes.

3. Meanwhile, place a large piece of wax paper on a work surface. Place fish fillets on wax paper, and cover with another piece. Use a flat-edged meat hammer to pound fish until they are very thin, about 1/4 inch. Check under the wax paper from time to time to make sure that fish is not tearing. Cut each piece in half to make 4 pieces.

1	**medium eggplant, sliced lengthwise into paper-thin slices**
2	**Tbsp extra-virgin olive oil, divided**
2	**cloves garlic, minced**
1	**cup chopped boxed tomatoes**
1	**cup strained boxed tomatoes**
2	**Tbsp freshly chopped basil**
2	**Tbsp pine nuts**
1/2	**tsp sea salt, divided**
1/8	**tsp freshly grated pepper**
	Dash crushed red pepper flakes
2	**boneless swordfish fillets (3/4 lb total)**

4. Top each piece of fish with thin layers of the eggplant slices. (If you have extra eggplant slices, reserve them as a garnish). Starting at the wide end, roll up fish, completely encasing eggplant. Use toothpicks or skewers to secure the rolls. Slowly remove lid from tomato sauce, and add rolls to simmering sauce. Cover, and cook for 10–15 minutes, turning once, or until fish is cooked through.

5. Transfer fish to a serving platter, remove skewers, and top with remaining sauce. Season with remaining 1/4 tsp salt, if desired. Serve remaining eggplant slices along the sides of the dish.

Healthy Living Tradition

A Turkish restaurateur told me that while he was working as a chef in Turkey, no one would hire him unless he knew at least 40 different eggplant dishes. Any less than 40 meant that you were a novice and didn't possess enough experience to work in fine restaurants. Take the Turkish challenge: try to collect 40 healthy eggplant recipes. Your body and your taste buds will be grateful.

Exchanges/Choices					
3 Vegetable	Calories	250	Sodium	405mg
2 Lean Meat	Calories from Fat	115	**Total Carbohydrate**	14g
2 Fat	**Total Fat**	13.0g	Dietary Fiber	4g
	Saturated Fat	2.1g	Sugars	7g
	Trans Fat	0.0g	**Protein**	19g
Serves 4	**Cholesterol**	35mg		
Serving Size: 1 bundle				

The famous Parisian restaurant Le Dome is celebrated for its exquisite fish dishes, which are filleted tableside. In this recipe, inspired by Le Dome's extensive seafood offerings, lemon or Dover sole fillets can be substituted for the whole fish. With this recipe by your side, you'll have an extraordinary main course in less than 15 minutes!

French Sole with Mushrooms and Asparagus

1. Heat 1 Tbsp extra-virgin olive oil in a large skillet over medium heat. Add mushrooms, cover, and cook until tender (about 10 minutes). Add asparagus, tomatoes, and *Herbes de Provence*. Cover, and cook for 5 minutes. Stir in lemon juice. Season with salt and pepper. Keep covered, and set aside.

2. Heat remaining 2 Tbsp extra-virgin olive oil in another large nonstick skillet over medium-high heat. Sprinkle fish with salt and pepper. Cook for about 2 minutes per side or until fish is opaque. Be careful not to overcook fish or it will become dry. Place fish on the bottom of one large or individual serving platters. Top and surround fish with sauce. Garnish with parsley.

3 **Tbsp extra-virgin olive oil, divided**
6 **oz fresh chanterelle mushrooms, trimmed and sliced**
1 **(1-lb) bag frozen asparagus spears, thawed and drained**
1 **cup peeled, seeded, and diced tomatoes**
1 **tsp Herbes de Provence (p. 277)**
  Juice of 1 lemon
  Grey sea salt or kosher salt, to taste
  Freshly ground pepper, to taste
4 **lemon or Dover sole fillets (1/4 lb each)**
2 **Tbsp fresh parsley, finely chopped**

Healthy Living Tradition

Grey sea salt is harvested by hand, organically produced, and unrefined. Its color comes from the fine grey clay of the ancient salt flats of Guerande in Brittany, France.

Exchanges/Choices		Calories	240	Sodium	110mg
2 Vegetable		Calories from Fat	110	Total Carbohydrate	9g
3 Lean Meat		Total Fat	12.0g	Dietary Fiber	3g
1 1/2 Fat		Saturated Fat	1.8g	Sugars	2g
		Trans Fat	0.0g	Protein	27g
Serves 4		Cholesterol	60mg		
Serving Size: 1 fillet					

This delicate fish dish is a surprising treat at the end of a long day. Turbot is found in both the Atlantic and Pacific oceans. It is also known as flounder, brill, fluke, and plaice. It is a member of the flat-fish family, which also contains sole and halibut. Any of those would make fine substitutions in this dish. This dish is of southern French origin, and it is important to note that *turbot* in French refers to a flavorful, diamond-shaped fish that is different from the Pacific flatfish known as turbot in the U.S.

Turbot with Watercress and Zucchini

1. Place flour on a plate. Add salt, pepper, and pepper flakes, and stir to combine. Dip turbot pieces in mixture to coat. Shake off excess. Transfer to a plate, and set aside.

2. Heat 2 Tbsp olive oil in a large, wide nonstick skillet over medium heat. Add fish. Brown on both sides (about 2 minutes per side). Add zucchini and squash. Pour in stock and lemon juice. Add thyme, cover, and allow to simmer for 5–10 minutes or until fish is cooked through and squash is tender. Remove and discard thyme.

3. Whisk balsamic vinegar with remaining 2 Tbsp olive oil in a small bowl. Toss watercress with balsamic vinegar dressing, taste, and season with salt and pepper as needed.

1/2 cup unbleached, all-purpose flour
1/4 tsp grey sea salt or other sea salt
Freshly ground pepper, to taste
Dash crushed red pepper flakes
4 (1/3 lb each) turbot fillets
4 Tbsp extra-virgin olive oil, divided
2 (1 lb each) bags frozen yellow and zucchini squash slices, thawed and drained
1 cup no-added-salt seafood stock
Juice of 1 lemon
2 sprigs fresh thyme
1 Tbsp balsamic vinegar
1 bunch fresh watercress, washed thoroughly and trimmed

4. Place watercress on the bottom of a large serving platter or divide among four individual plates. Place fish fillets on top of watercress, and scatter zucchini and squash around the sides.

Healthy Living Tradition

Watercress contains many important vitamins. To include more of this in your diet, try using watercress as a "bed" or accompaniment for fish dishes, as they do in North Africa, where watercress is also believed to heal skin maladies. It can also be added to sandwiches and used in place of lettuce in salads.

Exchanges/Choices					
1/2 Starch	Calories	360	Sodium	360mg
2 Vegetable	Calories from Fat	160	**Total Carbohydrate**	20g
3 Lean Meat	**Total Fat**	18.0g	Dietary Fiber	3g
3 Fat	Saturated Fat	2.7g	Sugars	3g
	Trans Fat	0.0g	**Protein**	29g
	Cholesterol	75mg		

Serves 4
Serving Size: 1 fillet

Baby squid are surprisingly simple to prepare. The tender texture of the calamari in this unique dish lends itself to a straight-forward cooking style.

Calamari Stuffed with Spinach

❁ Calamari Ripieni con Spinaci ❁

1. Heat 1 Tbsp olive oil in a large wide skillet over medium heat. Add onion, and sauté until golden (about 5 minutes). Add spinach, bread crumbs, salt, pepper, and red pepper flakes. Cook for 1 minute. Take mixture off heat, and allow to cool slightly.

2. Stuff calamari 3/4 of the way full with stuffing. Secure top with a toothpick.

3. Heat 1 Tbsp olive oil in a large frying pan over medium heat. Brown calamari on all sides. Add stock, cover, and simmer for 20–30 minutes on low until cooked through. Serve warm.

- 2 **Tbsp extra-virgin olive oil, divided**
- 1 **small yellow onion, finely chopped**
- 1 **cup frozen chopped spinach, thawed and drained well**
- 1/4 **cup plain bread crumbs**
- 3/4 **tsp salt**
  Freshly ground pepper, to taste
  Dash crushed red pepper flakes
- 1 **lb baby squid, tentacles removed and cleaned**
- 2 **cups fat-free, low-sodium vegetable or fish stock**

Healthy Living Tradition

Make your own fresh bread crumbs, a healthy and economical alternative to store-bought bread crumbs, by placing stale bread in the food processor and pulsing it on and off a few times.

Exchanges/Choices			
1/2 Starch			
1 Vegetable			
3 Lean Meat			
1/2 Fat			

Calories	225	**Sodium**	505mg
Calories from Fat	80	**Total Carbohydrate**	15g
Total Fat	9.0g	Dietary Fiber	3g
Saturated Fat	1.4g	Sugars	2g
Trans Fat	0.0g	**Protein**	21g
Cholesterol	265mg		

Serves 4
Serving Size: 3 oz

Tartines are open-faced sandwiches that are found in bistros all over France. They're elegant and simple, and the flavor combinations are endless. Any of the following salads will go well with this dish: *Corn, Tomato, Pea, and Dill Salad* (p. 185); *Romaine, Spinach, and Radicchio Salad* (p. 172); or *Chickpea, Tomato, and Tahini Salad* (p. 175).

Shrimp, Cucumber, and Boursin Tartines

1. Heat olive oil in a large skillet over medium-high heat. When olive oil begins to release its aroma, add shrimp, *Herbes de Provence*, and salt. Cook for 2–3 minutes per side or until shrimp are bright pink and cooked through.

2. For the bread slices, divide the round loaf into 8 equal parts. Cut loaf in half width wise first, and then divide each of the two pieces into quarters. Place bread slices on a work surface, and slather 1/2 tsp *boursin* on each slice.

3. Divide cucumber slices into four batches, and place a thin layer of cucumber on top of each bread slice, reserving extra, if necessary. Scatter shrimp on top of cucumber slices. Make a slit in the flesh of the lemon, twist it into an "S" shape, and place on top of tartine.

- 1 **Tbsp extra-virgin olive oil**
- 1 **lb shrimp, peeled and deveined**
- 1 **tsp Herbes de Provence (p. 277)**
- 1/2 **tsp kosher salt**
- 8 **(1-inch) slices country wheat French bread (such as boule, harvest)**
- 4 **tsp boursin cheese, at room temperature**
- 3/4 **lb English or Persian cucumbers, thinly sliced**
- 4 **thin lemon slices**

Healthy Living Tradition

Cool, mellow-tasting cucumbers are great to have on hand because they go with a multitude of dishes. Avoid the chemical wax coating on conventional cucumbers by buying organic ones when possible.

Exchanges/Choices			
1 Starch			
1 Vegetable			
2 Lean Meat			
1/2 Fat			

Calories	215	**Sodium**	540mg
Calories from Fat	65	**Total Carbohydrate**	21g
Total Fat	7.0g	Dietary Fiber	3g
Saturated Fat	1.3g	Sugars	2g
Trans Fat	0.0g	**Protein**	19g
Cholesterol	130mg		

Serves 8
Serving Size: 1 tartine

Paella is known as *arroz en paella* in its homeland of Spain. Original paella recipes consisted of rabbit, chicken, snails, and beans. The paella pans were rubbed in ash and cooked over orange wood. This "party in a pot" is said to be a descendant of Arabian *kabsah*, a similar dish originating in the Arabian Peninsula. Arabs introduced rice into southern Spain in the ninth century, along with spices like saffron.

Valencian Seafood Paella

1. Heat oil in a large wide skillet over medium heat. Add onion. Cook until golden brown (about 5 minutes). Add shrimp, squid, and fish to pan. Cook until barely opaque. Add rice and lima beans, and stir in saffron, paprika, garlic, and parsley. Pour the stock over the top of the mixture, and add salt. Increase the heat to high. Bring to a boil, reduce heat to low, and stir. Cook paella, uncovered, for 30–40 minutes or until all liquid is absorbed, stirring occasionally. When paella is done, allow to stand at room temperature for 10 minutes. Garnish with pimientos, and serve warm.

- 2 Tbsp extra-virgin olive oil
- 1 yellow onion, diced
- 1/4 lb jumbo shrimp, deveined and peeled
- 1 lb baby squid, cleaned, peeled, and sliced into rings
- 1/4 lb boneless white fish fillets (such as cod or swai)
- 2 cups medium-grain Spanish rice
- 1/2 lb frozen lima beans, thawed and drained
- Pinch high-quality saffron
- 2 tsp sweet paprika
- 1 clove garlic, chopped
- 2 Tbsp Italian parsley
- 5 cups low-sodium fish stock
- 1 tsp kosher salt
- 1/4 cup jarred pimiento peppers

Healthy Living Tradition

Paprika is high in vitamin C and contains a lot of antioxidants. In fact, by weight, paprika has even more vitamin C than lemon juice. Use paprika to flavor potatoes, rice, pasta, soups, and stews.

Exchanges/Choices	Calories	335	Sodium	405mg
3 Starch	Calories from Fat	45	**Total Carbohydrate**	51g
1 Vegetable	**Total Fat**	5.0g	Dietary Fiber	4g
2 Lean Meat	Saturated Fat	0.8g	Sugars	3g
	Trans Fat	0.0g	**Protein**	19g
Serves 8	**Cholesterol**	140mg		
Serving Size: 1 cup				

M'jadarah is a dish found in most Arab countries. It is a simple, delicious vegetarian main course.

Lentils and Rice

❋ *M'jadarah* ❋

1. In a medium saucepan, combine lentils, stock or water, salt, and pepper. Cook, uncovered, for 15 minutes over medium heat. Add rice and coriander, and mix well. Reduce heat to low, and cover. Cook until rice is tender and liquid is absorbed, 20–30 minutes.

2. While rice is cooking, heat olive oil over medium heat in a large frying pan. Add onion slices in a single layer. Sauté until dark golden and tender, about 10 minutes. Set aside.

3. When rice has finished cooking, fluff with a fork, and turn out onto a serving platter. Taste and add salt, if necessary. Pour oil and onions on top to garnish. Serve hot.

- **3/4 cup lentils, rinsed and sorted**
- **3 cups fat-free, low-sodium chicken or vegetable stock or water**
- **Salt, to taste**
- **Freshly ground pepper, to taste**
- **1 1/2 cups basmati rice**
- **1 tsp dried coriander**
- **2 Tbsp extra-virgin olive oil**
- **2 large onions, quartered and sliced**

Healthy Living Tradition

Incorporate beans and legumes into your favorite rice dishes for additional flavor and a nutritional boost.

Exchanges/Choices			
3 1/2 Starch	**Calories**	325	**Sodium** 255mg
1 Vegetable	Calories from Fat	45	**Total Carbohydrate** 59g
1/2 Fat	**Total Fat**	5.0g	Dietary Fiber 7g
	Saturated Fat	0.8g	Sugars 5g
	Trans Fat	0.0g	**Protein** 11g
Serves 6	**Cholesterol**	0mg	
Serving Size: 1/6 recipe			

Vegan dish

Traditional cassoulets (pronounced "cahs-oo-lay") are French country fare meant to be enjoyed on cold, blustery days. Taking advantage of leftovers, original versions contain duck breasts, pork, and sausage that are "stretched" by combining them with vegetables and topping with homemade bread crumbs. This is a healthy version that tastes great with the *Warm Goat Cheese Salad* (p. 173) and *Rustic Dinner Rolls* (p. 256) for a satisfying and authentic bistro-style meal at home. Keep in mind that dried lima beans require overnight soaking before proceeding with this recipe. Note that this recipe can be started on one day and finished on the day of serving, too.

Mixed Vegetable Cassoulet

1. Place lima beans in a large saucepan. Add water to cover, plus about 3 inches. Bring to a boil over high heat. Reduce heat to medium low, cover, and simmer for 1 hour or until tender. Drain and reserve.

2. Heat 2 Tbsp olive oil in a large, wide oven-proof skillet. Add onion and carrots, and sauté until onions are translucent. Stir in garlic, and allow to cook for 1 minute. Stir in cloves and bay leaf. Stir in lima beans, stock, and tomatoes. Increase heat to high, and bring to a boil, uncovered. Reduce heat to medium low, and simmer for 30 minutes, partially covered, or until beans and vegetables are tender and sauce has thickened.

3 cups dried lima beans, soaked overnight
4 Tbsp extra-virgin olive oil, divided
1 large yellow onion, diced
4 medium carrots, diced
4 cloves garlic, chopped
1/2 tsp ground cloves
1 Turkish or Mediterranean bay leaf
2 cups fat-free, low-sodium vegetable stock
1 cup diced tomatoes
2 cups coarse fresh bread crumbs from a baguette
1/2 cup freshly chopped parsley, divided
Salt, to taste
Freshly ground pepper, to taste

3. Preheat oven to 350°F. Toss bread crumbs with remaining 2 Tbsp olive oil and 1/4 cup parsley.

4. When cassoulet is ready, taste it, and add salt and pepper as needed. Stir in remaining 1/4 cup parsley. Mash beans slightly with a potato masher. (Recipe can be completed up until this step, brought to room temperature, and refrigerated. The next day, it can be topped with bread crumbs and baked for 30 minutes.)

5. Cover cassoulet with bread crumbs. Bake for 15 minutes or until golden.

Healthy Living Tradition

Want to regulate your digestion while feasting on international flavors? Try incorporating more beans and legumes into your diet. Lima beans are prized for their affordability and versatility, making them a vegetarian's best friend.

Exchanges/Choices	Calories		345	Sodium	125mg
2 1/2 Starch	Calories from Fat		70	**Total Carbohydrate**	53g
1 Vegetable	**Total Fat**		8.0g	Dietary Fiber	16g
1 Lean Meat	Saturated Fat		1.1g	Sugars	10g
1 1/2 Fat	Trans Fat		0.0g	**Protein**	17g
	Cholesterol		0mg		

Serves 8
Serving Size: 1 cup

Vegan dish

Variations on this dish are found throughout the Mediterranean. This is a flavorful and hearty dish that both vegetarians and meat eaters love.

Eggplant and Chickpea Stew

1. Heat 2 tsp olive oil in a large saucepan over medium heat. Add diced onions and garlic, and cook until onions are soft. Stir in the eggplant, chickpeas, cumin, cinnamon, coriander, tomatoes, salt, and pepper. Increase heat to high, and bring to a boil. Reduce heat to low, and cover the pot. Cook the stew for 45 minutes to 1 hour or until eggplant is very tender.

2. Meanwhile, heat remaining 2 tsp olive oil and add onion slices. Fry until golden, and remove from heat. When stew is finished, place in serving bowls and top with fried onions and cilantro.

- **4 tsp** extra-virgin olive oil, divided
- **2 medium** yellow onions, 1 diced and 1 sliced
- **3 cloves** garlic, minced
- **1 lb** eggplant, cubed
- **2 cups** canned no-salt-added chickpeas
- **1 tsp** ground cumin
- **1 tsp** ground cinnamon
- **1 tsp** ground coriander
- **1 (28-oz) can** no-salt-added diced or chopped tomatoes
- **1/4 tsp** salt
- **1/4 tsp** freshly ground pepper
- **1/4 cup** freshly chopped cilantro

Healthy Living Tradition

Many Middle Eastern and North African dishes rely on a large amount of onions and garlic. In addition to being affordable and plentiful, these wonderful ingredients pack in a lot of flavor without adding a ton of calories.

Exchanges/Choices					
1 Starch	**Calories**	270		**Sodium**	240mg
5 Vegetable	Calories from Fat	65		**Total Carbohydrate**	46g
1 Fat	**Total Fat**	7.0g		Dietary Fiber	12g
	Saturated Fat	0.8g		Sugars	17g
	Trans Fat	0.0g		**Protein**	11g
Serves 4	**Cholesterol**	0mg			
Serving Size: 1 1/2 cups					

Vegan dish

This tasty Turkish stew is like a garden harvest in a pot. It is worth searching out high-quality, organic vegetables whose tastes will take center stage in this recipe. Feel free to substitute whatever vegetables are fresh and available. If you choose to substitute frozen vegetables, thaw them, and add them to the recipe after the first 40 minutes of cooking, so that they will not become mushy.

Mixed Vegetable Stew ❄ *Turlu* ❄

1. Heat olive oil in a large saucepan over medium heat. Add onion, potatoes, okra, green beans, eggplant, and peas. Sauté until brown (about 5 minutes). Add mint, chili powder, salt, and pepper. Add enough water to cover vegetables. Increase heat to high, and bring to a boil. Reduce heat to low, cover, and simmer for 1 hour or until tender.

- 1 **Tbsp extra-virgin olive oil**
- 1 **yellow onion, diced**
- 3 **potatoes, peeled and cubed**
- 1/2 **lb okra, tops trimmed and sliced into rounds**
- 1/2 **lb green beans, trimmed**
- 1 **eggplant, chopped into 2-inch cubes**
- 1 **cup peas**
- 1 **tsp dried mint**
- 1 **tsp chili powder**
- 3/4 **tsp fine sea salt**
  Freshly ground pepper, to taste

Healthy Living Tradition

Double the quantities of this stew, and freeze half in single-size portions. You'll have a nutritious lunch or dinner for times when cooking isn't possible.

Exchanges/Choices			
1 1/2 Starch	**Calories**	205	
3 Vegetable	Calories from Fat	35	
1/2 Fat	**Total Fat**	4.0g	
	Saturated Fat	0.6g	
	Trans Fat	0.0g	
Serves 4	**Cholesterol**	0mg	
Serving Size: 1 1/2 cups			

Sodium	465mg
Total Carbohydrate	39g
Dietary Fiber	9g
Sugars	9g
Protein	7g

Vegan dish

A traditional recipe of the Spanish island of Majorca (about two hours south of Barcelona), this stew will easily get a variety of vegetables into your diet. Traditional accompaniments are freshly toasted bread, Manchego cheese, black olives, and salads. This stew can be served as a vegetarian main dish or as a side dish with seafood, chicken, or meat. It can be prepared a day ahead of time, and it freezes well.

Majorcan Vegetable Stew

❀ Sopa Mallorquinas ❀

1. Heat olive oil in a large stockpot or saucepan over medium heat. Add onion and bell pepper, and sauté until they begin to soften (about 5 minutes). Stir in garlic, cabbage, and cauliflower, and sauté for 5 more minutes or until cabbage begins to wilt. Add tomatoes, parsley, sage, rosemary, paprika, salt, pepper, and red pepper flakes. Stir. Add stock. Increase heat to high, and bring to a boil. Reduce heat to low, cover, and simmer for 30 minutes or until vegetables are soft. Remove lid, stir in spinach, and cook for 1–2 minutes or until spinach begins to wilt. Serve warm.

2 Tbsp extra-virgin olive oil
1 large yellow onion (about 1 cup), diced
1 green bell pepper (about 4 oz), chopped
4 cloves garlic, finely chopped
1 lb roughly chopped green cabbage
1 lb cauliflower florets
3 cups no-salt-added diced tomatoes
1/4 cup freshly chopped flat-leaf parsley
2 tsp chopped fresh sage
2 tsp chopped fresh rosemary
1 tsp high-quality paprika
1/2 tsp salt
1/2 tsp freshly ground pepper
   Pinch crushed red pepper flakes
3 cups fat-free, low-sodium vegetable stock
3 cups coarsely chopped fresh spinach leaves

Healthy Living Tradition

Many Mediterranean-style dishes incorporate a multitude of fresh vegetables. In recipes like this one, washing and chopping the vegetables takes more time than actually cooking the dish itself. Take a tip from housewives in the Mediterranean region: wash and chop your vegetables ahead of time. Many women sit at tables or cross-legged on tablecloths spread on the ground, chopping vegetables communally. This way they get to chat and enjoy one another's company while performing a mundane task.

Exchanges/Choices			
4 Vegetable • 1 Fat			

Calories	155	Sodium	435mg
Calories from Fat	55	Total Carbohydrate	24g
Total Fat	6.0g	Dietary Fiber	9g
Saturated Fat	0.8g	Sugars	12g
Trans Fat	0.0g	Protein	5g
Cholesterol	0mg		

Serves: 5 / Serving Size: 1 1/2 cups

Vegan dish

This is my version of a classic Italian dish, which is considered a Roman specialty. When I was just married and living in Rome, I prepared it weekly. Its simple, straightforward style and its sweet and piquant flavors make it a family favorite. For an authentic Roman experience, serve *Roman Spaghetti with Artichokes, Mint, and Garlic* (p. 74) as a first course and finish the meal with the *Mozzarella, Tomato, and Chickpea Salad* (p. 190).

Chicken, Tomato, and Pepper Stew
❊ *Pollo in Umido alla Romana* ❊

1. Heat olive oil in a large skillet over medium heat. Add chicken thighs. Brown for about 5 minutes on each side, turning once. Add bell peppers, and cook for about 5 minutes or until golden. Stir in garlic, and cook for 1 minute. Increase heat to high. Pour balsamic vinegar over the mixture. Allow to boil until vinegar has evaporated. Pour in stock and tomatoes, and stir. Stir in salt, pepper, and pepper flakes. When mixture comes to a boil, reduce heat to low, and cover. Simmer for 45 minutes or until peppers are tender and chicken is cooked through. Transfer to a serving plate and remove skin from chicken. Garnish with parsley. Serve hot.

1 1/2	Tbsp extra-virgin olive oil
3	lb chicken thighs
4	green bell peppers, cut into 1-inch strips
4	cloves garlic, minced
1/4	cup balsamic vinegar
1	cup fat-free, low-sodium vegetable stock
3	cups canned no-salt-added crushed tomatoes
1/2	tsp salt
1/2	tsp freshly ground pepper
	Pinch crushed red pepper flakes
4	Tbsp freshly chopped flat-leaf Italian parsley

Healthy Living Tradition

This sauce also tastes delicious when served on pasta, rice, pizza, or polenta. When making this dish, double the tomato and pepper amounts, and reserve the extra sauce to use on another dish later.

Exchanges/Choices	Calories	310	Sodium	315mg
3 Vegetable	Calories from Fat	135	Total Carbohydrate	14g
3 Lean Meat	Total Fat	15.0g	Dietary Fiber	4g
2 Fat	Saturated Fat	3.6g	Sugars	8g
	Trans Fat	0.0g	Protein	29g
Serves 6	Cholesterol	95mg		
Serving Size: 1 1/2 cups				

Tajines are dishes named after the vessel in which they are cooked. A *tajin* (with emphasis on the first syllable) is the word for a clay pot in Arabic. In Morocco, the word is pronounced *tajine* (with emphasis on the second syllable), and it refers to a clay pot with a cone-shaped lid in which such dishes are baked. Clay-pot cooking is great because it requires very little cooking oil to produce a great deal of flavor, making it a healthier cooking method. Also, seven is considered a lucky number in Moroccan culture, so seven vegetables are used in this dish. This recipe is strictly vegetarian. It is much more common to include meat in *tajines* in Morocco.

Moroccan Couscous with Vegetable Tajine

✹ Tajine Khodar bil Couscous ✹

1. Heat 1 tsp olive oil in a large, heavy pot over medium heat. Add onions. Sauté until translucent (about 5 minutes). Add 1/4 tsp salt, pepper, saffron, and turmeric. Stir to combine. Pour in boiling vegetable or chicken stock. Stir.

2. Add vegetables, cinnamon stick, and enough water to cover 3/4 of the vegetables. Stir. Increase heat to high, and bring to a boil, uncovered. Reduce heat to medium low, and simmer for 45 minutes, until vegetables are very tender and have broken down.

5 tsp extra-virgin olive oil, divided
2 yellow onions (about 8 oz total), chopped finely
3/4 tsp salt
Freshly ground pepper, to taste
1/2 tsp saffron
1 tsp turmeric
2 cups boiling vegetable or chicken stock (made with sodium-free bouillon granules)
1 lb carrots, peeled and chopped into 1-inch pieces
1/2 lb turnips, peeled and chopped into 1-inch pieces
1/2 lb artichoke hearts
1/2 lb zucchini, chopped into 1-inch pieces
1/2 lb eggplant, chopped into 1-inch pieces
1/2 lb potatoes, peeled and cut into large chunks
1/2 lb sweet potatoes, peeled and cut into large chunks
1 cinnamon stick
1 cup couscous

3. Ten minutes before *tajine* is finished, bring 1 1/4 cups water, 3 tsp olive oil, and 1/2 tsp salt to a boil in a medium saucepan over high heat. Take saucepan off heat, add couscous, stir, and cover with lid. Let stand for 10 minutes. Remove lid, fluff with fork, and stir in 1 tsp olive oil.

4. Serve in a large, shallow dish next to the *tajine*. When *tajine* is finished, remove cinnamon stick. Serve warm with 1/2 cup couscous.

Healthy Living Tradition

This seven-vegetable stew packs tons of much-needed vegetables into one dish. Think of ways you can introduce more vegetables into your favorite recipes to make them healthier.

Exchanges/Choices				
1 1/2 Starch	Calories	200	Sodium	285mg
2 Vegetable	Calories from Fat	30	Total Carbohydrate	38g
1/2 Fat	Total Fat	3.5g	Dietary Fiber	6g
	Saturated Fat	0.5g	Sugars	7g
	Trans Fat	0.0g	Protein	5g
Serves 8	Cholesterol	0mg		
Serving Size: 1 1/2 cups				

Vegan dish

This fresh spin on a French classic has a light, pleasant taste for the health conscious but will still satisfy hearty eaters. Cooked long-grain wild or brown rice is a great accompaniment to this dish.

French Fish Stew with Broccoli
❋ Blanquette de Poissons ❋

1. Place broccoli in a large saucepan, cover with water, and bring to a boil over high heat. Cook, uncovered, until tender (about 10 minutes). Drain, and set aside.

2. Place the carrot, onion, anise seeds, peppercorns, and salt in a large stockpot or saucepan. Add 4 cups water, and bring to a boil. Reduce heat to medium, and continue to cook, uncovered, for 15 minutes. Reduce heat to low, and add fish to the water. Cook, uncovered, for 5 minutes or until cooked through.

3. With a slotted spoon, carefully remove fish from the hot water. Strain remaining stock into another pot, and place over low heat. Combine lemon juice, lemon zest, and Dijon mustard. Stir into broth mixture. Increase heat to high, and cook until mixture is reduced by half. Place fish cubes and broccoli on a warm serving platter. Top with sauce. Serve hot.

1 1/4 **lb broccoli florets**
1 **medium carrot, peeled and trimmed**
1 **medium yellow onion, peeled and quartered**
1 **tsp anise seeds**
8 **whole peppercorns**
1 1/4 **tsp kosher salt**
2 **lb boneless firm fish (such as cod, haddock, salmon, rockfish) or a mix of fish, cut into 1 1/2-inch cubes**
1/4 **cup fresh lemon juice**
Zest of 1 lemon
1 **Tbsp Dijon mustard**

Healthy Living Tradition

Replacing traditional roux (butter and flour)-based sauces with lemon juice and Dijon mustard is a great way to thicken sauces and add flavor without bringing extra fat and calories to your dishes.

Exchanges/Choices		Calories	155	Sodium	580mg
1 Vegetable		Calories from Fat	15	**Total Carbohydrate**	6g
3 Lean Meat		**Total Fat**	1.5g	Dietary Fiber	3g
		Saturated Fat	0.3g	Sugars	2g
Serves 6		Trans Fat	0.0g	**Protein**	30g
Serving Size: 3 oz fish + 1/2 cup broccoli		**Cholesterol**	65mg		

Warm, rich beef stews evoke images of comfort and home. In many parts of the Mediterranean, beef was scarce and expensive. Beef-centered recipes were often "stretched" with vegetables and seasonings. This classic version contains beef for flavor and a medley of vegetables for additional texture and nutrition. If desired, serve with *Moroccan Country Bread* (p. 263).

Beef and Vegetable Stew

1. Heat olive oil in a large saucepan over medium heat. Add the onion, and stir. Sauté until translucent. Add beef, and brown on all sides. Add peas and carrots and green beans. Stir. Add stock, tomatoes, oregano, salt, and pepper. Stir. Add enough water to cover 3/4 of the mixture. Increase heat to high, bring mixture to a boil, and reduce heat to low. Stir, cover, and let simmer for 1 hour or until meat is tender. Taste and adjust seasonings, if necessary. Serve hot.

2 tsp extra-virgin olive oil
1 medium yellow onion (about 1/2 cup), finely chopped
1 lb beef cubes, cut into 1-inch pieces, for stewing
1 (16-oz) bag frozen peas and carrots, thawed
1 (16-oz) bag frozen green beans, thawed
2 cups fat-free, low-sodium vegetable, chicken, or beef stock
1/2 cup chopped or diced no-salt-added tomatoes
1 tsp oregano
1 tsp kosher salt
1/2 tsp freshly ground black pepper

Healthy Living Tradition

Make large quantities of this stew, and freeze it in individual serving sizes to eat when you're short on time.

Exchanges/Choices	Calories	165	Sodium	450mg
1/2 Starch	Calories from Fat	45	Total Carbohydrate	16g
1 Vegetable	Total Fat	5.0g	Dietary Fiber	6g
2 Lean Meat	Saturated Fat	1.2g	Sugars	6g
	Trans Fat	0.0g	Protein	16g
Serves 6	Cholesterol	35mg		
Serving Size: 1 1/2 cups				

Simple, Sensational Sides

Many people struggle with the idea of coming up with creative vegetable dishes that the whole family will love. In the Mediterranean region, this is never a problem. Traditional meals throughout the region consist of at least one (but often many more) cooked vegetables served as straightforward and uncomplicated side dishes. Made up of simply prepared vegetables, herbs, legumes, and pulses, they're both satisfying and healthful.

The dishes in this chapter were born out of the great agricultural centers throughout the region, which have been growing and cultivating crops since antiquity. Long before refrigeration and modern transportation were invented, only local in-season produce was available. Although the limited choices may seem daunting to many people nowadays, in ancient times people were accustomed to experimenting with produce and creating recipes out of single ingredients.

The Mediterranean lifestyle makes staying in touch with the seasons effortless. The open-air markets in the Mediterranean region were great centers of commerce, out of which numerous recipes and cultural traditions grew. Even today, strolling through maze-like streets lined with tables and crates stacked with bright, ripe, and perfectly plump produce, it is impossible not to become inspired by the freshness. The markets also provide convenient services to their patrons. For an extra fee, many vendors will chop vegetables and prepare them for cooking. They often share their secrets for delectable dishes with the produce at hand.

The open-air produce markets are set up daily or weekly in populous neighborhoods. Indoor markets provide people with staples and fill in the gaps between market days. Roadside produce stands are also popular with travelers. One of the

greatest times to drive through the Mediterranean countryside is during orange and lemon season. The citrus tree-studded orchards exude the intoxicating aroma of fragrant blossoms, which beckon visitors from miles away. Farmers sell their produce piled high in pretty pyramid shapes.

Many Mediterranean towns and villages celebrate the harvesting of various crops with festivals and carnivals that combine a particular vegetable prepared in both traditional and innovative ways with music, dancing, and games. In Italy, these festivals are known as *sagre*. On the Italian island of Sardinia, for example, there is an annual festival where fresh fennel takes center stage. At these festivals, humble plants become edible ambassadors. They are used to demonstrate important cultural Exchanges/Choices, promote the local economy, and create highly publicized parties, which draw people from all over the world. Each year, when new crops are cultivated, epicurean artisans skillfully pair them with hundreds of foods. After years of attending festivals like these, even ordinary people become adept at using vegetables in a multitude of ways.

Our modern American supermarkets are full of produce from all over the world, but many people do not know how to choose, clean, store, or cook with them. When cooking Mediterranean style, let seasonal availability and freshness help you decide which side dishes to prepare. Take excursions to farmer's markets and orchards, and stock up on high-quality produce. This will help you and your family stay in sync with which foods are seasonal. Most farmer's markets and organic grocers also offer charts to help shoppers determine which crops are in season. Use the recipes in this chapter to explore new ways of incorporating delectable vegetables into your diet.

Across the Mediterranean region, fennel is celebrated for its mildly sweet flavor, culinary versatility, nutritional benefits, and budget-friendly price. Fennel is an herbaceous plant that originated in the Mediterranean region, where it has been used since 3000 BCE. The ancient Romans used dried fennel seeds to preserve foods. Fennel bulbs can be eaten raw, pickled, or cooked. The fennel stalks, which resemble celery, can be added into slow simmering stocks or stews for additional flavor.

Braised Fennel with Orange Sauce

❋ Finocchi all'Arancia ❋

1. Heat oil in a large skillet over medium heat. Add the fennel bulbs and seeds, and cook fennel for 5 minutes on each side or until golden. Stir in the parsley, salt, pepper, stock, and orange juice. Increase heat to high, and bring to a boil. Reduce heat to low, cover, and simmer for 10–20 minutes or until fennel is tender and most of the liquid has reduced. Transfer to a serving platter. Sprinkle with cheese. Serve warm.

- 2 Tbsp extra-virgin olive oil
- 3 lb fennel, bulbs quartered and stalks reserved for another use
- 1 tsp fennel seeds, crushed in a mortar
- 1 cup freshly chopped Italian parsley
- 1/2 tsp salt
- 1/2 tsp freshly ground black pepper
- 1 cup fat-free, low-sodium vegetable stock
- 1/2 cup freshly squeezed orange juice
- 1/4 cup grated Parmigiano Reggiano cheese

Healthy Living Tradition

In the Mediterranean region, many people munch on raw fennel the way Americans enjoy crunchy celery sticks.

Exchanges/Choices				
3 Vegetable	Calories	115	Sodium	330mg
1 Fat	Calories from Fat	55	Total Carbohydrate	15g
	Total Fat	6.0g	Dietary Fiber	6g
	Saturated Fat	1.1g	Sugars	6g
Serves 6	Trans Fat	0.0g	Protein	4g
Serving Size: 1/2 cup	Cholesterol	0mg		

Vegan dish

Green beans contain vitamins A and C and folate. This is a quick and tasty way to serve them.

Stewed Green Beans

❀ *Lubiya Matboukh* ❀

1. Heat olive oil in a medium saucepan over medium heat. Add onion. Sauté until translucent (3–5) minutes. Stir in garlic, and cook for 1 minute. Stir in tomatoes, thyme, salt, and pepper. Bring to a boil over high heat. Add green beans, stir, and reduce heat to low. Simmer for 10–15 minutes or until green beans are tender. Spoon onto a serving platter, and top with fresh parsley.

1	Tbsp extra-virgin olive oil
1	small yellow onion, diced
4	cloves garlic, chopped
1 3/4	cups diced tomatoes
1	tsp fresh thyme, finely chopped
1	tsp salt
	Freshly ground black pepper, to taste
1	lb French-style green beans, ends trimmed
1	Tbsp fresh parsley, finely chopped

Healthy Living Tradition

In Mediterranean cultures, children are always involved in preparing food. Kitchen tasks give children an increased sense of responsibility and teach them cooking skills, which will enable them to make healthy meals for themselves. Trimming green beans was one of my kitchen tasks as a young child. If you have children in your family, think about ways to get them involved.

Exchanges/Choices	Calories	45	Sodium	295mg
1 Vegetable	Calories from Fat	20	Total Carbohydrate	7g
1/2 Fat	Total Fat	2.0g	Dietary Fiber	2g
	Saturated Fat	0.3g	Sugars	2g
Serves 8	Trans Fat	0.0g	Protein	2g
Serving Size: 1/2 cup	Cholesterol	0mg		

Vegan dish

This traditional Lebanese dish combines roasted eggplant, yogurt, and pine nuts. Its silky, velvety texture and mellow taste make it an excellent alternative to mashed potatoes. When served with pita bread or crudités, this dish can be a healthy and tasty appetizer.

Eggplant with Yogurt, Tahini, and Pine Nuts

1. Place a colander inside a bowl. Add yogurt. Set in the refrigerator for 6 hours or overnight.

2. Preheat broiler. Prick the eggplants in a few places with a knife, and place them on a baking sheet. Broil the eggplants for 20 minutes or until they are soft and wilted. Remove from the broiler. Allow to cool slightly. When cool enough to handle, peel them with your fingers and slice off the tops. Place in a fine sieve or colander, and press them gently to remove the juices.

- 1 **cup whole-milk yogurt, drained overnight**
- 2 **lb eggplant**
- 2 **Tbsp tahini**
- 1/2 **tsp kosher salt**
- 1/4 **tsp freshly ground black pepper**
- 1 **Tbsp olive oil**
- 2 **Tbsp pine nuts**

3. Transfer to a medium bowl. Stir in drained yogurt and tahini. Taste, and season with salt and pepper, if necessary.

4. Heat olive oil in a small frying pan over medium heat. Add pine nuts, and toast quickly over low heat. Remove from heat when golden.

5. Spoon mixture onto a serving dish. Pour pine nuts and oil over the top. Serve warm or at room temperature.

Healthy Living Tradition

In Turkey, the mark of a good cook is whether he or she knows how to make more than 40 eggplant dishes. Since eggplant is a healthy ingredient, you can never have too many!

Exchanges/Choices			
2 Vegetable	Calories	95	Sodium	130mg
1 Fat	Calories from Fat	55	Total Carbohydrate	9g
	Total Fat	6.0g	Dietary Fiber	3g
	Saturated Fat	1.3g	Sugars	3g
Serves 8	Trans Fat	0.0g	Protein	3g
Serving Size: 1/4 cup	Cholesterol	5mg		

Eggplant is low in carbohydrates and contains calcium, phosphorus, potassium, and thiamin. Luckily, Mediterranean cuisine is full of delicious eggplant recipes that were developed to create diversity during the eggplant harvest season, when people had to eat a lot of it. This dish is an attractive side dish or appetizer. It can be made a day ahead of time, stored in the refrigerator, and reheated in the oven before serving.

Mediterranean Eggplant

1. Cut tops off eggplants. Cut eggplants in half lengthwise, making two boat shapes. With a corer or grapefruit spoon, carefully remove the flesh from the eggplant, leaving a very thin layer next to the skin. Cut the flesh into small cubes and set aside.

2. Fill a medium pot 3/4 full with water. Bring to a boil over high heat. Add tomatoes to boiling water, and allow to boil for a few minutes or until skin begins to split. Remove tomatoes from boiling water and drain. Place them in a bowl of cold water and ice to stop cooking. When tomatoes are cool enough to handle, peel and dice them.

- 1 **lb baby eggplants (about 4, at 4 oz each)**
- 5 **ripe Roma tomatoes**
- 3 **Tbsp extra-virgin olive oil, divided**
- 1 **Tbsp black Kalamata or Gaeta olives, pitted**
- 1 **tsp capers, rinsed and drained**
- 2 **cloves garlic, minced**
- 2 **Tbsp freshly chopped basil leaves**
- 1/2 **tsp kosher salt**
- 1/4 **tsp freshly ground black pepper**
- 1 **Tbsp freshly grated Parmesan cheese**

3. Heat 2 Tbsp olive oil in a large skillet over medium-high heat. Add eggplant cubes. Allow to cook for about 3 minutes per side or until they begin to soften and change color. Add tomatoes, olives, capers, garlic, basil, salt, and pepper. Stir. Reduce heat to medium low, cover, and simmer for 10–20 minutes or until vegetables are tender.

4. Meanwhile, heat the oven to 400°F. Oil a baking dish (large enough to fit the 8 eggplant boats in a single layer) with remaining 1 Tbsp olive oil. Arrange eggplant boats in baking dish.

5. When vegetables have finished cooking, stir in Parmesan. Stuff the eggplant boats up to the tops with the vegetable mixture. Bake, uncovered, for 45 minutes or until eggplant is tender and mixture is golden.

Healthy Living Tradition

Eggplant is a low-carb culinary canvas that marries well with many flavors. Try using it in place of potatoes in some of your recipes.

Exchanges/Choices	Calories	150	Sodium	295mg
3 Vegetable	Calories from Fat	100	**Total Carbohydrate**	13g
2 Fat	**Total Fat**	11.0g	Dietary Fiber	4g
	Saturated Fat	1.7g	Sugars	5g
Serves 4	Trans Fat	0.0g	**Protein**	2g
Serving Size: 2 eggplant halves	**Cholesterol**	0mg		

This popular Mediterranean side dish is enjoyed in late spring, when baby artichokes are at their peak. In addition to their mellow, buttery flavor, fresh baby artichokes have a tender texture and offer elegant presentation. If you've never worked with fresh artichokes before, don't be intimidated. The steps to preparing them are simple, and after cooking them once you'll be a pro. If baby artichokes are not in season, substitute reduced-sodium canned artichoke hearts or frozen ones.

Baby Artichokes with Herb Sauce

1. Soak the artichokes in water to clean. Drain and repeat until water is clear. Peel away the outside leaves of the bottom half of the artichokes. Cut off the top quarter of the artichoke. At this point, the artichoke should look like a flower, and the tough, dark leaves should all be removed, leaving only lighter colored, tender leaves. If tough, dark green leaves remain, peel those off as well.

2. Add juice of 1 lemon to a bowl full of cold water. Add artichokes to water to avoid discoloration.

12 baby artichokes
2 lemons, juiced, divided
2 Tbsp extra-virgin olive oil
1 Tbsp Dijon mustard
1/4 tsp salt
1/8 tsp freshly ground black pepper
1 Tbsp fresh mint, finely chopped
1 Tbsp fresh dill, finely chopped
1 Tbsp fresh flat leaf parsley, finely chopped

3. Bring a large pot of water to a boil, and add cleaned artichokes. Bring to boil over high heat. Reduce heat to medium low, and simmer 15–20 minutes or until tender. Drain artichokes. Set aside.

4. Place remaining lemon juice, olive oil, and mustard in a blender. Whip together to form a vinaigrette. Stir in salt, pepper, mint, dill, and parsley. Pour dressing over artichokes. Serve warm or at room temperature.

Healthy Living Tradition

Artichokes are a delightful addition to many dishes. Keep frozen artichokes on hand to add to salads, pasta, and rice dishes.

Exchanges/Choices	Calories	115	Sodium	295mg
2 Vegetable	Calories from Fat	65	**Total Carbohydrate**	12g
1 Fat	**Total Fat**	7.0g	Dietary Fiber	8g
	Saturated Fat	1.0g	Sugars	1g
Serves 4	Trans Fat	0.0g	**Protein**	3g
Serving Size: 3 artichokes	**Cholesterol**	0mg		

In the North African countries along the Mediterranean, it is the artichoke bottoms, not the hearts, which are coveted. This simple recipe combines the soft texture of the artichokes with the chewy texture of slightly *al dente* rice. The flowery artichoke flavor is boosted by a topping of sharp cheese. This side dish is a succulent accompaniment to *Poached Sea Bass with Tomatoes and Herbs* (p. 117), *Chicken Thighs with Tomato-Tarragon Sauce* (p. 96), and *Roasted Cod with Tomatoes, Zucchini, and Olives* (p. 116). This dish can be made a day ahead of time, stored in the refrigerator, and reheated before serving. Artichoke bottoms can be found in Mediterranean and Middle Eastern grocery stores in jarred and frozen varieties.

Stuffed Artichoke Bottoms

1. Heat 1 Tbsp olive oil in a medium saucepan with a tight-fitting lid over medium heat. Add rice, and toast on all sides. Pour in 3/4 cup vegetable stock, increase heat to high, and bring to a boil. Stir, reduce heat to low, and simmer for 10–15 minutes or until liquid is absorbed and rice is *al dente*.

2. Meanwhile, grease the bottom of an oven-proof dish with 1 Tbsp olive oil.

3. When rice is ready, remove the lid, and stir in diced red pepper, salt, pepper, and lemon juice. Stuff artichoke bottoms with rice mixture, and sprinkle the tops of each evenly with cheese. Arrange stuffed artichokes in the oven-proof dish.

4. Pour remaining 3/4 cup vegetable stock into the bottom of the dish. Cover with aluminum foil. Bake for 45 minutes or until artichokes and rice are tender and cheese is melted.

2 Tbsp extra-virgin olive oil, divided
1 cup Arborio or Egyptian rice
1 1/2 cups fat-free, low-sodium vegetable stock, divided
1 jarred roasted red pepper, diced
Salt, to taste
Freshly ground pepper, to taste
Juice of 1/2 lemon
8 artichoke bottoms
1 oz freshly grated Romano cheese

Healthy Living Tradition

Stuffed vegetables are as visually appealing as they are healthful. By using vegetables as edible containers, you'll be able to add variety, style, and nutrients to your meals without a lot of effort.

Exchanges/Choices		Calories	130	Sodium	185mg
1 Starch		Calories from Fat	40	**Total Carbohydrate**	19g
1 Fat		**Total Fat**	4.5g	Dietary Fiber	2g
		Saturated Fat	1.1g	Sugars	1g
Serves 8		Trans Fat	0.0g	**Protein**	3g
Serving Size: 1 each		**Cholesterol**	5mg		

Given the popularity of potatoes in the modern Mediterranean region, it's hard to believe that they're not native to the area. Potatoes are a product of the New World and were brought to Europe by the Spaniards. They were incredibly unpopular and were served as gruel, prison food, and feed for animals. It wasn't until Marie Antoinette wore a potato blossom in her fashionable hair that the French people began incorporating them into their diets. This rustic, homey version of a potato cake is a guiltless pleasure. It's the perfect complement for dishes of roasted meat, fish, or poultry.

Potato-Artichoke Torte

1. Preheat oven to 350°F. Oil an 8-inch cake pan with 1 Tbsp olive oil. Place potatoes in one layer on the bottom of the baking pan. Scatter artichokes along the top. Sprinkle salt, pepper, garlic, parsley, cheese, and bread crumbs over the top. Drizzle remaining 1 Tbsp olive oil over the top. Bake 30–45 minutes or until the tops of the potatoes are golden.

2 Tbsp extra-virgin olive oil, divided
1 lb (about 2) Yukon Gold potatoes, peeled and cut into 1/4-inch rounds
1 (14-oz) can artichoke hearts, rinsed and drained
  Kosher salt, to taste
  Freshly ground pepper, to taste
4 cloves garlic, minced
1/4 cup fresh parsley, finely chopped
2 Tbsp Romano cheese
2 Tbsp plain bread crumbs

Healthy Living Tradition

Combining green vegetables like artichokes and spinach with potatoes is popular in Italy. In addition to making the dish more healthful, it inspires even those who avoid green vegetables to eat and love them.

Exchanges/Choices		Calories	200	Sodium	310mg
2 Starch		Calories from Fat	70	**Total Carbohydrate**	27g
1 Fat		**Total Fat**	8.0g	Dietary Fiber	4g
		Saturated Fat	1.4g	Sugars	3g
Serves 4		Trans Fat	0.0g	**Protein**	5g
Serving Size: 2-inch slice		**Cholesterol**	5mg		

Roasted potatoes are a common street snack in North African cities. The combination of Moroccan spices and olive oil enhances the sweet flavors of the potato. Serve this side dish with *Grilled Grouper with Moroccan Dipping Sauce* (p. 119) or *Eggplant and Chickpea Stew* (p. 134).

Spice-Dusted Sweet Potatoes

1. Preheat oven to 400°F. Prick sweet potatoes with a fork, and place in the middle of the oven. Bake for about 1 hour or until potatoes are soft when pressed.

2. Halve sweet potatoes by splitting lengthwise and making crisscross cuts in the flesh. Drizzle olive oil evenly over the flesh of the four halves. Sprinkle the *Moroccan Ras El Hanout Spice Mix* and pepper over each one. Serve hot.

- **2 sweet potatoes (about 1 lb each), scrubbed**
- **2 Tbsp extra-virgin olive oil**
- **1 Tbsp Moroccan Ras el Hanout Spice Mix (p. 284)**
- **1 Tbsp freshly ground pepper**

Healthy Living Tradition

The sweet potato has a low glycemic index value, which means that eating them won't raise blood glucose levels as high as eating other potatoes. For a healthy variation, try replacing the potatoes in your favorite recipes with sweet potatoes.

Exchanges/Choices		Calories	235	Sodium	430mg
2 1/2 Starch		Calories from Fat	65	**Total Carbohydrate**	40g
1 Fat		**Total Fat**	7.0g	Dietary Fiber	7g
		Saturated Fat	1.0g	Sugars	12g
Serves 4		Trans Fat	0.0g	**Protein**	4g
Serving Size: 1/2 sweet potato		**Cholesterol**	0mg		

Vegan dish

It's amazing what the flavor of a few simple herbs can do to enhance the taste of potatoes. Whenever I bring this recipe to a potluck, people can't stop commenting on it. They're relieved and thrilled to learn how easy it is to make at home.

Oven-Roasted Herb Potatoes

❋ *Patatas fee al forn* ❋

1. Preheat oven to 425°F. Oil a large baking dish or cookie sheet with 1 tsp olive oil. Add potatoes, garlic, salt, dill, mint, and lemon juice to baking dish. Toss well to combine. Drizzle remaining olive oil over potatoes, and mix well. Bake, uncovered, for 45 minutes to 1 hour or until potatoes are tender.

2 Tbsp extra-virgin olive oil, divided
4 (2 1/2-inch diameter) Yukon Gold, Idaho, or Russet potatoes, scrubbed and cut into 2-inch cubes
8 cloves garlic, chopped
1 1/2 tsp fine sea salt
1 Tbsp dried dill
1 Tbsp dried mint
1/4 cup fresh lemon juice

Healthy Living Tradition

Roasting vegetables is a simple and healthy Mediterranean tradition. Asparagus, tomatoes, peppers, eggplant, onions, zucchini, carrots, and parsnips can all be prepared the same easy way. Mix and match your favorite vegetables to create new family favorites.

Exchanges/Choices					
1 Starch	**Calories**	100	**Sodium**	450mg	
1/2 Fat	Calories from Fat	30	**Total Carbohydrate**	16g	
	Total Fat	3.5g	Dietary Fiber	2g	
	Saturated Fat	0.5g	Sugars	1g	
Serves 8	Trans Fat	0.0g	**Protein**	2g	
Serving Size: 1/2 cup	**Cholesterol**	0mg			

Vegan dish

Years ago, the idea of eating mashed potatoes without butter and cream would have made me cringe. Once I tasted this delicious Tunisian recipe, however, I discovered a tastier, healthier way of enjoying potatoes. The combination of buttery golden baby potatoes, citrusy lemon, flowery cilantro, and zippy dill provides intense flavor. This dish tastes great with *Chicken Thighs with Tomato-Tarragon Sauce* (p. 96) and *Salmon-Stuffed Cabbage Leaves* (p. 120).

Herb and Olive Oil Mashed Potatoes

1. Place potatoes in a large pot, and cover with water. Bring to a boil over high heat, reduce heat to medium, and cook, uncovered, for 10–15 minutes or until tender. Drain. Add lemon juice and olive oil, and begin mashing by hand or with an electric mixer. When mixture is smooth and creamy, stir in lemon zest, cilantro, dill, salt, and pepper. Serve warm.

- **10 baby golden potatoes (about 1 lb each), scrubbed and quartered**
- **1/4 cup freshly squeezed lemon juice**
- **2 Tbsp extra-virgin olive oil**
- **Zest of 1 lemon**
- **1/4 cup cilantro, finely chopped**
- **1/4 cup dill, finely chopped**
- **1/2 tsp sea salt or kosher salt**
- **1/4 tsp freshly ground black pepper**

Healthy Living Tradition

If you're not serving mashed potatoes immediately, you can keep them warm by placing them in a metal bowl and covering them with aluminum foil. Place the bowl inside a saucepan with 1/4 inch boiling water at the bottom (make sure the bowl doesn't touch the bottom of the saucepan).

Exchanges/Choices		Calories	120	Sodium	205mg
1 Starch		Calories from Fat	40	**Total Carbohydrate**	18g
1 Fat		**Total Fat**	4.5g	Dietary Fiber	2g
		Saturated Fat	0.6g	Sugars	1g
Serves 6		Trans Fat	0.0g	**Protein**	2g
Serving Size: 1/2 cup		**Cholesterol**	0mg		

Vegan dish

Okra has been present in Egypt since antiquity. Now, versions of this stew are served throughout the Middle East. Sometimes it is served with beef or veal cubes.

Stewed Okra and Tomatoes

❀ *Bamya Matbukh* ❀

1. Heat olive oil in a medium saucepan over medium heat. Add the onion, stir, and sauté until translucent. Add okra, and stir to combine. Add stock, tomatoes, oregano (wild thyme can be substituted), salt, and pepper to taste. Bring to a boil over high heat; then reduce heat to low. Stir, cover, and let simmer for 20 minutes or until okra is tender. Serve hot.

- **2 tsp extra-virgin olive oil**
- **1 medium yellow onion, finely chopped**
- **3 cups fresh or frozen okra (baby okra can be left whole; otherwise slice into 1/4-inch rounds)**
- **2 cups fat-free, low-sodium vegetable, chicken, or beef stock**
- **1/2 cup diced tomatoes**
- **1 tsp dried oregano**
- **1 tsp salt**
- **Freshly ground black pepper, to taste**

Healthy Living Tradition

Making vegetable-based stews is a succulent way to increase vegetable consumption. Use this recipe as a base for any kind of vegetables you choose to prepare.

Exchanges/Choices			
2 Vegetable			

Calories	50	Sodium	440mg
Calories from Fat	15	Total Carbohydrate	8g
Total Fat	1.5g	Dietary Fiber	3g
Saturated Fat	0.3g	Sugars	4g
Trans Fat	0.0g	Protein	2g
Cholesterol	0mg		

Serves 6
Serving Size: 1/2 cup

Vegan dish

Lentils have been a powerful trading commodity since antiquity. This is a simple, delicious vegan dish to enjoy with warm pita bread, couscous, or rice.

Moroccan Lentils with Stewed Tomatoes

1. Place lentils in a medium saucepan, and add water to cover. Bring to a boil over high heat, reduce to low, and simmer, covered, for 30 minutes or until tender. Drain and reserve. (This step may be done a day ahead of time.)

2. Combine lentils, tomatoes, onion, coriander, salt, and pepper in a large saucepan. Add 1 cup water, and place over high heat. Bring to a boil, and reduce heat to low. Simmer, covered, for 20–30 minutes or until lentils are tender. Add cilantro. Stir. Serve hot.

1 **cup brown lentils, rinsed and sorted**
1 **cup chopped canned or boxed no-salt-added tomatoes**
1 **medium yellow onion (about 1/2 cup), chopped**
1 **tsp dried coriander**
1 **tsp kosher salt**
1/4 **tsp freshly ground black pepper**
1/4 **cup fresh cilantro, finely chopped**

Healthy Living Tradition

Make a double batch of lentils, and keep half reserved before combining them with other ingredients in this recipe. They make a great protein-rich, low-fat addition to soups, salads, and sauces.

Exchanges/Choices		Calories	90	Sodium	250mg
1 Starch		Calories from Fat	0	Total Carbohydrate	16g
		Total Fat	0.0g	Dietary Fiber	6g
Serves 8		Saturated Fat	0.0g	Sugars	2g
Serving Size: 1/2 cup		Trans Fat	0.0g	Protein	7g
		Cholesterol	0mg		
Vegan dish					

These are a healthy alternative to poppers. This recipe makes a great appetizer or buffet item because it can be prepped a day in advance and baked at the last minute and, if necessary, served at room temperature.

Stuffed Orange and Yellow Mini Peppers

1. Preheat oven to 450°F. Slice the tops off mini peppers, and remove seeds.

2. Combine 2 Tbsp olive oil, bread, garlic, parsley or cilantro, capers, salt, and pepper in a food processor. Pulse to form a thin paste. If the mixture is runny, add more bread. If it is too thick, add 1 tsp water at a time.

3. Carefully stuff each mini pepper with the filling without puncturing the pepper. Fill each pepper to the top. Coat a small baking or loaf pan with 1 Tbsp olive oil. Lay peppers in a single layer in the bottom of the pan. Drizzle with remaining 1 Tbsp olive oil.

4. Bake for 10–15 minutes on each side, until the peppers are soft and slightly browned. Serve warm or at room temperature.

12   sweet orange and yellow mini peppers (about 3 inches long)
4   Tbsp extra-virgin olive oil, divided
2   (3-inch) pieces day-old Italian or French bread with crusts, broken into 1-inch pieces
2   cloves garlic
1/2   cup fresh parsley or cilantro leaves, finely chopped
1   tsp capers, rinsed and drained
1/4   tsp kosher salt
1/8   tsp freshly ground pepper

Healthy Living Tradition

Bright, colorful foods are not only appealing to the eye, they're also good for the body. Try to incorporate orange and yellow peppers, cantaloupe, carrots, and yellow squash into your diet.

Exchanges/Choices		Calories	130	Sodium	190mg
1/2 Starch • 1 Vegetable		Calories from Fat	80	Total Carbohydrate	11g
1 1/2 Fat		Total Fat	9.0g	Dietary Fiber	1g
		Saturated Fat	1.3g	Sugars	1g
Serves 6		Trans Fat	0.0g	Protein	2g
Serving Size: 2 mini peppers		Cholesterol	0mg		

Vegan dish

Mozzarella, Tomato, and Chickpea Salad, 190
Israeli Orange and Honey-Glazed Chicken with Almonds, 94

Corn, Tomato, Pea, and Dill Salad, 185
Southern French-Style Herb-Roasted Turkey, 106

Tunisian Fish Couscous, 115
Tomato and Pepper Salad, 179

Cool Carrot Purée with Bell Pepper Sticks, 20
Roasted Cod with Tomatoes, Zucchini, and Olives, 116

Bruschetta with Artichoke Purée and Roasted Red Peppers, 27
Sicilian Swordfish and Eggplant Bundles, 124

Spanish Gazpacho Soup Shooters, 57
Valencian Seafood Paella, 130

Stuffed Orange and Yellow Mini Peppers, 158
*Spicy Israeli Tomato Spread ,*33
Spice-Dusted Sweet Potatoes, 153

Apple, Date, and Raisin Phyllo Strudel, 212
Mini Mixed Berry Crostata, 200
Fresh Figs with Raspberry Purée, 229

This dish is a popular Italian side dish that also works well as an appetizer when used to top crostini or as a first course when used to dress pasta. It is traditionally served alongside grilled or roasted meat and poultry dishes.

Stewed Cannellini Beans with Tomatoes and Sage

❋ *Fagioli al'uccelletto* ❋

1. Heat 1 Tbsp oil in a wide skillet over medium heat. Add garlic. Cook until it begins to release its aroma. Add beans with liquid from can, sage, tomatoes, and pepper. Stir to combine, reduce heat to low, and cover. Simmer 5–10 minutes or until most of the liquid is absorbed. Mash lightly with a fork, and transfer to serving plate. Drizzle the remaining olive oil over the top, and serve warm.

- 2 Tbsp extra-virgin olive oil, divided
- 2 cloves garlic, minced
- 1 (15-oz) can low-sodium cannellini beans, undrained
- 5 fresh sage leaves, finely chopped
- 1/4 cup strained tomatoes or low-sodium crushed tomatoes
- 1/4 tsp freshly grated black pepper

Healthy Living Tradition

Beans are a great source of protein and fiber. Fiber is an essential part of a healthy diet.

Exchanges/Choices			
1 Starch	Calories	150	Sodium	35mg
1 Lean Meat	Calories from Fat	70	Total Carbohydrate	15g
1 Fat	Total Fat	8.0g	Dietary Fiber	4g
	Saturated Fat	1.0g	Sugars	1g
	Trans Fat	0.0g	Protein	5g
Serves 4	Cholesterol	0mg		
Serving Size: 1/2 cup			

Vegan dish

Most of the chestnuts sold in the U.S. are harvested in early October in Italy. Chestnuts were originally native to the U.S., but countless groves died from blight in the early 20th century. Chestnuts were always an important culinary staple for Native Americans, Italians, and the French. Over the years, they have become a fall and winter favorite. Roasted chestnuts are sold on the streets throughout great Italian and French cities. Around the base of the *Sacre Coeur* cathedral in Paris and along the *Via del Corso* in Rome, the fragrant chestnut smell lends a homey, comforting scent to the air from October to December.

Cider-Glazed Chestnut, Butternut Squash, and Cauliflower Medley

1. Heat the oil in a large skillet over high heat. Add the squash and cauliflower (if using frozen, add during next step). Reduce heat to medium. Sauté, uncovered, for 5–7 minutes. Stir in the apple, chestnuts, and sage. Slowly add the stock and cider. Increase heat to medium high, and bring to a simmer. Scrape up the brown bits in the bottom of the pan. Simmer for 10–15 minutes or until vegetables are tender and most of the liquid is absorbed. Season with salt and pepper to taste.

2 **Tbsp olive oil**
6 **oz butternut squash, peeled and diced into 1-inch pieces**
8 **oz fresh cauliflower florets (or frozen, thawed, and drained)**
1 **large Granny Smith apple, peeled, cored, and diced into 1-inch pieces**
8 **oz whole roasted or steamed chestnuts, peeled**
1 **Tbsp fresh sage, chopped finely**
1/2 **cup fat-free, low-sodium chicken or vegetable stock**
1/4 **cup apple cider**
1/4 **tsp kosher salt**
Freshly ground black pepper, to taste

Healthy Living Tradition

Mediterranean meal patterns include both cooked and fresh vegetables at every meal. Roasting vegetables is a popular cooking method because vegetables do not lose as many nutrients during cooking, it is easy to do, and it also concentrates their flavors.

Exchanges/Choices		Calories	160	Sodium	135mg
1 Starch • 1/2 Fruit		Calories from Fat	45	Total Carbohydrate	27g
1 Fat		Total Fat	5.0g	Dietary Fiber	3g
		Saturated Fat	0.8g	Sugars	9g
Serves 6 / Serving Size: 1/2 cup		Trans Fat	0.0g	Protein	2g
		Cholesterol	0mg		

Vegan dish

This mixture is known as *peperonata* in Italy and is a typical garnish for roasted and grilled meats.

Mixed Pepper Medley

1. Heat olive oil in a large, wide skillet over medium heat. Add peppers, and brown on each side. Stir in garlic, and cook for 1 minute. Add olives, reduce heat to low, and cover. Cook for 20 minutes or until peppers are tender. Stir in vinegar. Taste, and add salt if needed.

3 Tbsp extra-virgin olive oil
2 lb mixed red, yellow, and green bell peppers, cut into thin strips
6 cloves garlic, minced
1/4 cup green olives, pitted and diced
2 Tbsp balsamic vinegar
Salt, to taste

Healthy Living Tradition

One of the easiest ways to ensure a healthy diet is to incorporate a variety of multicolored produce into your meals.

Exchanges/Choices	Calories	160	Sodium	135mg
3 Vegetable	Calories from Fat	110	**Total Carbohydrate**	14g
2 Fat	**Total Fat**	12.0g	Dietary Fiber	3g
	Saturated Fat	1.6g	Sugars	7g
Serves 4	Trans Fat	0.0g	**Protein**	2g
Serving Size: about 1 cup	**Cholesterol**	0mg		

Vegan dish

This is one of the most simple and satisfying Mediterranean recipes to make. Hot, tender, vegetables seasoned with roasted garlic, lemon, olive oil, and *Herbes de Provence* make healthy eating a pleasure. Best of all, this recipe requires very little attention while cooking, leaving you free to do other things. Serve these vegetables with grilled, roasted, or pan-fried fish, meat, or poultry.

Mediterranean Roasted Vegetables

1. Preheat oven to 425°F. Coat a 9 × 13-inch baking dish with olive oil. Add eggplant, zucchini, and red peppers. Toss to combine. Sprinkle *Herbes de Provence*, salt, and pepper on top. Place garlic, peeled side down, in the middle of the pan. Squeeze lemon juice over the top. Roast, uncovered, for 45 minutes or until vegetables are tender.

2. Remove from oven. Remove garlic from pan. When garlic is cool enough to handle, squeeze cloves out and stir them into the vegetables. Stir to combine. Serve warm.

2 **Tbsp extra-virgin olive oil**
1 **medium (8–9 inches) eggplant, cut into 1-inch pieces**
2 **zucchini (1/2 lb), cut into 1-inch rounds**
2 **red peppers (6 oz each), cut into 1-inch pieces**
1 **Tbsp Herbes de Provence (p. 277)**
1 **tsp kosher salt**
1/2 **tsp freshly ground black pepper**
1 **head garlic, top peeled off, left whole**
   Juice of 1 lemon

Healthy Living Tradition

The next time you're making a roast, try adding the healthy vegetables from this recipe in addition to, or instead of, traditional potatoes and carrots.

Exchanges/Choices	Calories		55	Sodium	245mg
1 Vegetable	Calories from Fat		30	**Total Carbohydrate**	6g
1/2 Fat	**Total Fat**		3.5g	Dietary Fiber	2g
	Saturated Fat		0.5g	Sugars	2g
Serves 8	Trans Fat		0.0g	**Protein**	1g
Serving Size: 1/2 cup	**Cholesterol**		0mg		

Vegan dish

Grilled vegetables are used in a multitude of ways in Italian kitchens. From antipastos to pastas and accompaniments for second courses, you'll find them everywhere. This dish works very well for buffets.

Grilled Italian Vegetables

1. Place eggplant on a large baking tray, and sprinkle with some salt. Let stand at room temperature to draw out the bitter juices. Drain, rinse well, and pat dry.

2. Combine balsamic vinegar, olive oil, garlic, 1/2 tsp salt, 1/4 tsp pepper, and basil in a small bowl. Set aside.

3. Place whole peppers over an open flame on a gas grill or broil under the broiler until blackened and blistered. Place in paper lunch bags, and seal shut. In a few minutes, open the bags carefully (steam will escape and can burn), remove peppers, peel off the skin, and cut into slices.

1	small, firm eggplant, cut into 1/2-inch thick slices
	salt, to taste
1/4	cup balsamic vinegar
1/4	cup extra-virgin olive oil
2	cloves garlic, finely minced
1/4	tsp freshly ground pepper
1/4	cup fresh basil, finely chopped
2	large red peppers
4	small zucchini, trimmed and cut in half

4. Preheat broiler or grill. Place eggplant and zucchini on a large baking tray. Broil or grill until golden and tender on both sides. When done, stir in peppers, pour dressing over, and mix. Serve hot or at room temperature.

Healthy Living Tradition

Grilling is one of the least fattening ways of preparing vegetables. Try grilling vegetables in large batches and storing them in the refrigerator in individual containers. Use them throughout the week to top pizzas, to add to pastas and soups, or to serve as fast side dishes.

Exchanges/Choices		Calories	95	Sodium	225mg
2 Vegetable		Calories from Fat	65	**Total Carbohydrate**	9g
1 Fat		**Total Fat**	7.0g	Dietary Fiber	2g
		Saturated Fat	1.0g	Sugars	5g
Serves 8		Trans Fat	0.0g	**Protein**	1g
Serving Size: 1 cup		**Cholesterol**	0mg		

Vegan dish

This delicious and nutritious dish makes a unique side or vegetarian main dish.

Bean, Lentil, and Spinach Skillet

1. Place lentils in a saucepan, and cover with water. Bring to a boil over high heat. Reduce heat to medium. Cook, uncovered, for 20–30 minutes or until tender.

2. Heat 1 Tbsp olive oil in a large wide skillet. Add onion. Stir often until golden and caramelized. Set aside.

3. Add remaining 2 Tbsp olive oil to another large skillet. Add the spinach, and cover. Cook for 3–5 minutes or until spinach becomes tender. Stir in garlic. Cook until it releases its aroma. Add chickpeas and stir. When lentils are ready, drain and stir into mix, along with the lemon juice. Taste, and season with salt and pepper. Top with caramelized onions, if desired, and serve hot.

1/2 cup lentils, sorted and rinsed
3 Tbsp extra-virgin olive oil, divided
1 large yellow onion, sliced
1/2 lb fresh spinach
3 cloves garlic, minced
1 (15 oz) can no-salt-added chickpeas, drained and rinsed
2 Tbsp lemon juice
Salt, to taste
Freshly ground black pepper, to taste

Healthy Living Tradition

Even if you're not a vegetarian, replacing a few servings of meat per week with high-fiber legume dishes like this one will get you on track with your fiber intake.

Exchanges/Choices					
1 Starch	Calories	215	Sodium	35mg
1 Vegetable	Calories from Fat	70	Total Carbohydrate	28g
1 Lean Meat	Total Fat	8.0g	Dietary Fiber	9g
1 1/2 Fat	Saturated Fat	1.1g	Sugars	5g
	Trans Fat	0.0g	Protein	10g
	Cholesterol	0mg		

Serves 6
Serving Size: 1/2 cup

Vegan dish

Sunny Salads

I know many wonderful home cooks and chefs who adore food. Most of them have no difficulty deciding what to make for dinner or creating new recipes for their restaurants. Where people tend to get stuck, however, is on salads. Have you ever noticed how few salad options there are on most restaurant menus? Even when there are a lot of choices, salads are often laden with heavy dressings and contain fattening meats and fried ingredients. Home cooks usually end up serving the same salads over and over. Because dietary guidelines promote eating five to thirteen servings of fruits and vegetables a day, we should all broaden our salad repertoire in order to enjoy our meals and our health to the fullest.

If you are one of the many people who finds yourself in a salad rut, don't despair. Mediterranean salads are a cause for celebration. They are beautiful to look at, easy to prepare, and taste delicious. Containing everything from lettuces and herbs to fruits, vegetables, grains, pulses, dairy, eggs, and cheeses, the salads of the region are truly spectacular. By learning how to create these salads, you'll be able to enjoy a healthier, more varied diet. Here are some tips:

1. Include a salad at each meal.

2. Vary the kinds of salad you eat daily.

3. Only use the freshest in-season produce in salads.

4. Use extra-virgin olive oil, vinegars, and citrus juice for dressings.

5. Be creative in combining fruits with your salad—tomatoes, after all, are a fruit.

6. Experiment with stretching salads with leftover ingredients to create quick, healthy meals.

Another important component of serving Mediterranean-style salads is to coordinate the serving of the salad with the customs of the recipe's country of origin. There are four basic types of salads in the Mediterranean. The "after the main event" salads, the "appetizer and meal-accompanying" salads, the "stretched" salads, and the trendy "restaurant" salads featured in this book all make delicious additions to any meal.

The southern European Mediterranean areas in France, Italy, Spain, and Greece serve salads after the main course, by themselves, to cleanse the palate. These are known as "after the main event" salads. These salads are not meant to be eaten alone or as a meal. Their function is to simply provide fresh fruits and vegetables and to prepare the palate for the next course of the meal, which usually consists of cheeses and/or fruit and dessert. The *Orange, Asparagus, and Avocado Salad* (p. 168), *Pear and Radicchio Salad with Pistachios* (p. 170), *Red Cabbage Salad* (p. 171), and *Romaine, Spinach, and Radicchio Salad* (p. 172) are all examples of the "after the main event" salad. These salads are light, easy to prepare, and simple enough for every day, yet special enough for entertaining.

The second kind of Mediterranean salad is found in North African and Middle Eastern countries, such as Morocco, Tunisia, Algeria, Libya, Egypt, Turkey, Lebanon, and Israel. These countries all serve salads as part of appetizers before the meal or with the meal at intimate family affairs. The *Carrot, Date, and Orange Salad* (p. 176), *Egyptian Country Salad* (p. 178), and the *Mixed Algerian Salad* (p. 180) are all examples of appetizer or accompanying salads. These salads are great for adding variety to your everyday meals.

Another kind of salad, which I refer to as the "stretched" salad, is often prepared in homes around the Mediterranean. One of the tenets of the Mediterranean kitchen is never to throw anything away. People are very resourceful and take great pride at transforming leftover morsels into culinary masterpieces. Because lunch is typically the largest, most important meal of the day in the region, dinners tend to be simple, healthful affairs, especially when eaten at home. "Stretched" salads combine seasonal produce with leftover croutons, fish, chicken, poultry, seafood, beans, or pulses to make a more substantial, yet still light, meal. In various regions in Italy, for example, there is a salad called *insalata del lunedi*, which is made from leftover morsels of meat and other items from the Sunday roast. In this book, the *Shepherd's Salad* (p. 181), *Fattoush Salad* (p. 182), and *Sicilian Salad with Potatoes* (p. 184) are perfect examples of the culinary potential of leftovers. These salads are great for saving time and money while stretching your creativity.

Trendy "restaurant" salads have become popular in the Mediterranean region, much like in the U.S. One difference that is unique to the Mediterranean area, however, is that salad bars often consist of trays full of distinct, already-prepared salads. Even fast-food American-style hamburger and pizza chains in places like Italy and Egypt offer these kinds of salads, which are popular with the locals. Diners simply go to deli counters inside restaurants and order a sampling (some places let you take them yourself) of fresh, interesting salads that are eaten before the meal. The *Corn, Tomato, Pea, and Dill Salad* (p. 185), *Cucumber, String Bean, and Olive Tapenade Salad* (p. 186), *Lebanese Bulgur, Tomato, and Cucumber Salad* (p. 177), *Marinated Eggplant Salad* (p. 187), *Moroccan Salad Trio* (p. 188), and *Mozzarella, Tomato, and Chickpea Salad* (p. 190) are all examples of trendy "restaurant" salads that are a cinch to make at home. These salads also make popular potluck dishes and work great for buffets.

So the next time you're in a salad rut, open the pages of this chapter. Whichever salad you choose to create will add a burst of fresh flavors to your meal and diversity to your diet.

This salad is bright and beautiful. The combination of oranges and tomatoes offers a nice tangy complement to the rich avocado and asparagus flavors.

Orange, Asparagus, and Avocado Salad

1. Place asparagus in a pot of boiling water over high heat. Reduce heat to low. Simmer until asparagus is tender. Drain, and place in a bowl of ice-cold water.

2. Divide lettuce evenly among six salad bowls or plates.

3. Combine orange, tomato, and avocado in a medium bowl.

4. Whisk together olive oil, vinegar, salt, and pepper in a small bowl until combined.

5. Drain asparagus, and add to orange mixture. Pour dressing over orange mixture. Stir gently to combine. Spoon mixture on top of romaine lettuce on plates. Serve.

1 **bunch fresh asparagus, trimmed (about 8 oz)**
4 **oz romaine lettuce, cut into bite-size pieces**
1 **large orange, trimmed and cut into segments**
1 **large ripe tomato, cut into 8 equal pieces**
1 **avocado, peeled, pitted, and diced**
2 **Tbsp extra-virgin olive oil**
1 **Tbsp red wine vinegar**
1/4 **tsp kosher salt**
1/4 **freshly ground pepper**

Healthy Living Tradition

Although avocados originated in Latin America, they are now extremely popular in Europe. They contain a good amount of vitamin K, potassium, and folate and a ton of dietary fiber. They are also a great source of healthier unsaturated fats.

Exchanges/Choices		Calories	110	Sodium	90mg
1/2 Carbohydrate		Calories from Fat	70	**Total Carbohydrate**	9g
1 1/2 Fat		**Total Fat**	8.0g	Dietary Fiber	4g
		Saturated Fat	1.2g	Sugars	5g
Serves 6		Trans Fat	0.0g	**Protein**	2g
Serving Size: 3/4 cup		**Cholesterol**	0mg		

Vegan dish

Sicily is known for its beautiful, lush orange groves, which produce some of the world's most fragrant oranges. First introduced by the Arabs during their rule of the island, the oranges flourished in the ashes along the base of Mt. Etna. Look for the sweetest oranges possible for this recipe. When possible, use Sicilian blood oranges. Their red color gives festive flair to this sumptuous salad.

Orange and Fennel Salad
❋ *Insalata di Finocchi ed Arancie* ❋

1. Cut stalks off fennel, and reserve for use in stocks or soups, or discard. Remove bruised leaves. Slice off ends of the bulb bases, cut into quarters, and slice into thin slices horizontally. Place in a salad bowl. Add oranges and parsley, and toss lightly to combine.

2. Whisk orange juice, lemon juice, and olive oil together, and season with salt and pepper. Pour over the salad. Serve immediately.

2 **large fennel (anise) bulbs (about 1 1/2 lb total)**
2 **large oranges (about 1 lb total), peeled and sliced into segments**
4 **Tbsp fresh parsley, chopped**
  Juice of 1 orange
  Juice of 1 lemon
2 **Tbsp extra-virgin olive oil**
1/4 **tsp salt**
  Freshly ground pepper, to taste

Healthy Living Tradition

Fresh fennel is popular in the Mediterranean and is used for both culinary and medicinal uses. Dried fennel seeds are used to freshen breath and as a digestive aid from the Mediterranean region to India. Fennel tea is also made by boiling 1 tsp fennel seeds and straining it. It is usually enjoyed at night, after a meal.

Exchanges/Choices		Calories	95	Sodium	130mg
1/2 Fruit		Calories from Fat	40	**Total Carbohydrate**	13g
1 Vegetable		**Total Fat**	4.5g	Dietary Fiber	3g
1 Fat		Saturated Fat	0.6g	Sugars	8g
		Trans Fat	0.0g	**Protein**	1g
Serves 6		**Cholesterol**	0mg		
Serving Size: 1/2 cup					

Vegan dish

Italians usually follow their meals with a salad and end them with fruit. This unique salad combines both courses in one. Orange blossom water is made from the oil of fresh orange blossoms. It is used throughout the Mediterranean in dressings and sweets. It is sold in specialty stores and in Mediterranean and Middle Eastern markets. If you cannot find it, substitute orange juice.

Pear and Radicchio Salad with Pistachios

❀ Insalata di Pere, Radicchio, e Pistacchi ❀

1. Place radicchio in a large bowl or on a serving platter. Arrange pear slices on top of radicchio. Pour 1/2 of lemon juice on top of pears.

2. Make dressing by combining remaining lemon juice, sugar, and orange blossom water in a small bowl. Whisk in the olive oil until blended, and season with salt and pepper.

3. Pour dressing over salad, and top with pistachios.

1 head radicchio, chopped into bite-size pieces
2 medium D'Anjou pears, peeled, cored, and sliced into sixths
1/4 cup lemon juice, divided
1 tsp sugar
1 tsp orange blossom water or orange juice
2 Tbsp extra-virgin olive oil
Salt, to taste
Freshly ground pepper, to taste
1/4 cup shelled pistachios, roughly chopped

Healthy Living Tradition

In the spring, winter, and fall, when tomatoes aren't at their peak, try using other fruits in your salads. Strawberries are great in spring, lemons and oranges work great in winter, and apples and pears are perfect during fall.

Exchanges/Choices		Calories	160	Sodium	15mg
1 Fruit		Calories from Fat	100	**Total Carbohydrate**	17g
2 Fat		**Total Fat**	11.0g	Dietary Fiber	3g
		Saturated Fat	1.4g	Sugars	9g
Serves 4		Trans Fat	0.0g	**Protein**	3g
Serving Size: about 1/2 cup		**Cholesterol**	0mg		

Vegan dish

This salad combines the great flavors and colors of red cabbage, carrots, artichokes, and tomatoes. It's a rainbow of flavors in a bowl. Serve it in place of traditional coleslaw.

Red Cabbage Salad

1. Combine cabbage, carrots, artichoke hearts, and tomato in a large bowl.

2. In a small bowl, whisk together mustard, vinegar, and lemon juice. Slowly add olive oil to the mixture, whisking to incorporate thoroughly. Season with salt and pepper.

3. Toss salad with dressing to coat. Serve immediately or store salad and dressing separately in the refrigerator, and serve on the following day.

1 (11-oz) head red cabbage, cored and leaves shredded

2 carrots, peeled and shredded

1 (6-oz) jar artichoke hearts, rinsed and drained

1 Roma tomato, diced

1 tsp Dijon mustard

1 Tbsp balsamic vinegar
Juice of 1/2 lemon

3 Tbsp extra-virgin olive oil
Kosher salt, to taste
Freshly ground pepper, to taste

Healthy Living Tradition

Many people skip fresh salads with their meals because they're a hassle to make. To make salads hassle free, keep them in your refrigerator undressed, so that they will stay fresh and be ready for you when you need them.

Exchanges/Choices		Calories	145	Sodium	180mg
2 Vegetable		Calories from Fat	90	**Total Carbohydrate**	12g
2 Fat		**Total Fat**	10.0g	Dietary Fiber	3g
		Saturated Fat	1.4g	Sugars	5g
Serves 4		Trans Fat	0.0g	**Protein**	2g
Serving Size: 1 cup		**Cholesterol**	0mg		

Vegan dish

Mixing various types of salads together makes a more fulfilling salad. Here, crunchy romaine, tender baby spinach, and crisp, bitter radicchio blend well. Serve this salad as a light finale to a meal that features hearty sauces and stews.

Romaine, Spinach, and Radicchio Salad

1. Combine romaine, spinach, and radicchio in a large salad bowl.

2. Place olive oil in a small bowl. Vigorously whisk in vinegar until dressing is incorporated and thick. Season with salt and pepper. Pour over salad.

1 1/3 cups shredded romaine lettuce
1 1/3 cups baby spinach
1 1/3 cups shredded radicchio
3 Tbsp extra-virgin olive oil
3 Tbsp balsamic vinegar
Salt, to taste
Pepper, to taste

Healthy Living Tradition

You'll be much more inclined to eat salad if you wash it ahead of time. I like to wash my lettuce in a salad spinner. Then, I store it between paper towels wrapped in plastic or stored in a plastic bag. It stays fresh in the refrigerator for a week and is ready whenever I need it.

Exchanges/Choices		Calories	105	Sodium	10mg
1 Vegetable		Calories from Fat	90	**Total Carbohydrate**	4g
2 Fat		**Total Fat**	10.0g	Dietary Fiber	1g
		Saturated Fat	1.4g	Sugars	2g
Serves 4		Trans Fat	0.0g	**Protein**	1g
Serving Size: 1 cup		**Cholesterol**	0mg		

Vegan dish

Salads topped with warm goat cheese are French bistro classics. Luckily, they're easy and inexpensive to make at home. This salad tastes great at suppertime with a soup like the *Potato and Herb Soup* (p. 62) or *Traditional Minestrone* (p. 61).

Warm Goat Cheese Salad

1. Pour lemon juice into a bowl. Whisk in mustard, sugar, and olive oil. Taste, and add salt and pepper.

2. In a large bowl, combine lettuce and carrots. Mix well.

3. With a sharp knife, slice the goat cheese into 8 rounds. Heat a skillet over medium heat, and warm goat cheese on both sides. Cook for 1–2 minutes until warm and golden.

4. Divide lettuce leaves evenly among four plates. Top with cheese and dressing.

- 4 **Tbsp lemon juice**
- 1 **tsp Dijon mustard**
- 1/2 **tsp sugar**
- 2 **Tbsp extra-virgin olive oil**
  Salt, to taste
  Freshly ground pepper, to taste
- 3 **cups mixed green lettuce or mesclun**
- 1 **cup shredded carrots**
- 3 **oz reduced-fat goat cheese**

Healthy Living Tradition

Adding some shredded leftover chicken or meat and chickpeas turns this delicious side salad into a great weeknight meal or lunch.

Exchanges/Choices		Calories	75	Sodium	85mg
1 Vegetable		Calories from Fat	55	**Total Carbohydrate**	4g
1 Fat		**Total Fat**	6.0g	Dietary Fiber	1g
		Saturated Fat	1.4g	Sugars	2g
Serves 6		Trans Fat	0.0g	**Protein**	2g
Serving Size: 1/6 recipe		**Cholesterol**	0mg		

Cucumber is a wonderful vegetable. This classy Italian sorbet is like a frozen salad to be used as an opener for meals on a hot summer day. I like to serve it in a scoop in the middle of a salad plate surrounded by tomato slices and topped with a few shredded carrots. It has all of the flavors of a normal salad, but in an unexpected, elegant way.

Cucumber Sorbet

❀ *Sorbetto di cetrioli* ❀

1. Place cucumber pieces and olive oil in the food processor. Pulse on and off to purée. Stop often, and scrape down the sides. Add ice cubes one at a time, and continue to pulse until mixture resembles a sorbet. Serve immediately, or freeze until ready to use. If sorbet is frozen, break up crystals with a fork before serving.

1 **cucumber, seeded and cubed**
1 **Tbsp extra-virgin olive oil**
  About 24 ice cubes

Healthy Living Tradition

One of the "tricks" of spa chefs is to serve healthful foods in unexpected ways to delight their guests' eyes and taste buds at the same time without adding unwanted calories and fat. Look at some of the healthiest dishes you like to prepare and think of new ways to prepare and present them.

Exchanges/Choices	Calories	40	Sodium	0mg
1 Vegetable	Calories from Fat	30	**Total Carbohydrate**	3g
1/2 Fat	**Total Fat**	3.5g	Dietary Fiber	0g
	Saturated Fat	0.5g	Sugars	1g
Serves 4	Trans Fat	0.0g	**Protein**	0g
Serving Size: 1/2 cup	**Cholesterol**	0mg		

Vegan dish

Tender chickpeas, crunchy parsley, and fresh, juicy tomatoes provide a perfect balance of textures in this salad. This dish works well for buffet-style dining and picnics. It can also be added to couscous for a light, vegetarian meal.

Chickpea, Tomato, and Tahini Salad

❀ *Salata Hommus bil Tomatum wa Tahina* ❀

1. Combine chickpeas, tomatoes, and parsley on a medium serving platter.

2. Pour lemon juice into a medium bowl, and add tahini (can be purchased in the international section in most supermarkets), salt, and pepper. Whisk mixture vigorously to incorporate. Pour dressing over salad. Mix well to combine. Serve at room temperature.

2 cups canned chickpeas, rinsed and drained
1 cup cherry or grape tomatoes
1/4 cup fresh parsley, finely chopped
Juice of 1 lemon
2 Tbsp tahini (sesame paste)
1/4 tsp salt
Freshly ground pepper, to taste

Note: To make this salad ahead of time, simply keep the dressing and the salad separate and refrigerate one day ahead of time. Before serving, pour dressing over salad, and mix well.

Healthy Living Tradition

In many countries around the Mediterranean, salads like this one are made in advance and served in large buffets or salad bars. For a light lunch or dinner, people combine three or four small servings of various salads.

Exchanges/Choices					
1 Starch	Calories	120	Sodium	195mg
1 Lean Meat	Calories from Fat	35	Total Carbohydrate	17g
	Total Fat	4.0g	Dietary Fiber	5g
	Saturated Fat	0.5g	Sugars	4g
Serves 6	Trans Fat	0.0g	Protein	6g
Serving Size: 1/2 cup	Cholesterol	0mg		

Vegan dish

This refreshing salad is a Moroccan favorite that makes the most out of three widely used ingredients. In the countryside where orange orchards are common, families press their own orange oil to make orange blossom water. In the U.S., orange blossom water can be found in specialty stores. Even children will love the unique combination of soft and crunchy textures and sweet and sour tastes in this salad.

Carrot, Date, and Orange Salad
❋ Salata bil Jazar, Tamr, wa Bortuan ❋

1. Arrange romaine on the bottom of a large serving dish. Scatter carrots on top of lettuce. Arrange oranges on top of carrots. Arrange dates around the top.

2. Make dressing by whisking orange juice, lemon juice, orange blossom water, and pepper together in a small bowl. Drizzle over the salad. Serve immediately.

4 cups chopped romaine lettuce
2 medium carrots, peeled and grated
1 navel orange, peeled and cut into segments
1/4 cup pitted dates
  Juice of 1 orange
  Juice of 1 lemon
1 tsp orange blossom water
  Freshly ground pepper, to taste

Healthy Living Tradition

Follow nature's lead when making healthy changes to your diet. A handy rule is "if it grows together, it goes together." In-season fruits and vegetables can be combined in many delicious and unique ways.

Exchanges/Choices	Calories	40	Sodium	15mg
1/2 Fruit	Calories from Fat	0	Total Carbohydrate	9g
	Total Fat	0.0g	Dietary Fiber	2g
Serves 8	Saturated Fat	0.0g	Sugars	7g
Serving Size: 3/4 cup	Trans Fat	0.0g	Protein	1g
	Cholesterol	0mg		
Vegan dish				

This classic salad originated in Lebanon, where it is a nutritious lunch or picnic item that is often included in everyday family meals. The flavors in this salad continue to develop while the salad is stored in the refrigerator, so it actually benefits from being made a day in advance. To eat, place a few spoons of *tabouleh* on a lettuce leaf, wrap it up, and eat it with your fingers.

Lebanese Bulgur, Tomato, and Cucumber Salad

❊ *Tabouleh* ❊

1. Pour bulgur into a large bowl. Add water to cover, plus 2 inches. Let stand for 1 hour. (This step can be done a day in advance.)

2. Mix bulgur with olive oil, lemon juice, and lime juice. Add salt and pepper. Add diced vegetables and chopped herbs. Stir. Taste and adjust seasonings if necessary.

3. Refrigerate for 1–12 hours. Serve with large whole romaine leaves.

1/2 **cup medium bulgur wheat**
1/4 **cup extra-virgin olive oil**
1/4 **cup lemon juice**
1/4 **cup lime juice**
1 **tsp salt**
  Freshly ground pepper, to taste
2 **English cucumbers, diced**
4 **Roma tomatoes, diced**
1 **red onion, diced**
3/4 **cup fresh parsley, chopped**
1/4 **cup fresh mint, chopped**
1 **head romaine lettuce, leaves cleaned and rinsed**

Healthy Living Tradition

When you're trying to reduce your caloric or carbohydrate intake, try wrapping sandwich and other fillings in lettuce instead of bread. You get additional crunch and fiber in your meal.

Exchanges/Choices		Calories	115	Sodium	300mg
1/2 Starch • 1 Vegetable		Calories from Fat	65	Total Carbohydrate	13g
1 Fat		Total Fat	7.0g	Dietary Fiber	3g
		Saturated Fat	1.0g	Sugars	4g
Serves 8		Trans Fat	0.0g	Protein	2g
Serving Size: 1/2 cup		Cholesterol	0mg		

Vegan dish

This is the most commonly served salad in North Africa. The vegetables used in making it vary depending on the time of year and availability. Be sure to finely dice the vegetables to achieve the proper texture.

Egyptian Country Salad

❋ *Salata Baladi* ❋

1. Place cucumber, carrot, parsley, green bell pepper, and tomato in a large bowl.

2. Whisk oil, lime peel, lime juice, salt, pepper, cumin, and chili powder together in a medium bowl. Pour dressing over salad, and toss to combine.

1 **cucumber, diced**
1 **carrot, shredded**
1 **bunch flat-leaf parsley, finely chopped**
1 **green bell pepper, diced**
1 **large tomato, diced**
1/4 **cup olive or expeller-pressed corn oil**
Grated peel and juice of 2 limes
Salt, to taste
Freshly ground black pepper, to taste
Dash cumin
Dash chili powder

Healthy Living Tradition

In North Africa, herbs are treated not only as flavor enhancers, but as base ingredients like lettuce. For variety, try fresh cilantro, parsley, arugula, and other herbs in place of other lettuces.

Exchanges/Choices		Calories	105	Sodium	20mg
1 Vegetable		Calories from Fat	80	**Total Carbohydrate**	6g
2 Fat		**Total Fat**	9.0g	Dietary Fiber	2g
		Saturated Fat	1.3g	Sugars	3g
Serves 6		Trans Fat	0.0g	**Protein**	1g
Serving Size: 1/2 cup		**Cholesterol**	0mg		

Vegan dish

This popular salad can be served as an appetizer or accompaniment to grilled and roasted meats. Try making it during the summer, when peppers and tomatoes are at their peak.

Tomato and Pepper Salad

1. Preheat broiler or grill. Grill peppers until blistered (about 5–10 minutes), turning often. Remove from oven or grill, and place in paper bags for 5 minutes. Fold tops of the paper bags over, and tape them shut to enclose steam. Allow peppers to stand for 10 minutes or up to 1 hour. After the 10 minutes have passed, carefully release the steam from the paper bags. (This step can be done a day ahead of time.)

2. Peel the skin off the peppers, cut off the tops, and slice into 1/2-inch strips. Place in a salad bowl, and add capers, parsley, and garlic.

3. In a small bowl, whisk together the olive oil and vinegar. Add tomato to the bowl, and drizzle over peppers. Stir gently to coat. Taste, and season with salt and pepper as needed. Serve at room temperature.

2 large yellow bell peppers
2 large red bell peppers
2 large green bell peppers
2 Tbsp capers
2 Tbsp freshly chopped Italian parsley
1 clove garlic, chopped
2 Tbsp extra-virgin olive oil
1 Tbsp balsamic vinegar
1 large tomato, thinly sliced
Kosher salt, to taste
Freshly ground black pepper, to taste

Healthy Living Tradition

Bell peppers are low in calories and carbohydrate, but high in flavor. The vibrant range of colors in which they are available will bring beauty to your table.

Exchanges/Choices		Calories	95	Sodium	90mg
3 Vegetable		Calories from Fat	45	**Total Carbohydrate**	13g
1/2 Fat		**Total Fat**	5.0g	Dietary Fiber	3g
		Saturated Fat	0.7g	Sugars	7g
Serves 6		Trans Fat	0.0g	**Protein**	2g
Serving Size: 1/2 cup		**Cholesterol**	0mg		

Vegan dish

Some of the recipes that were introduced to the U.S. from France, Spain, and Italy were actually of North African descent. Years of trade and exchange as well as foreign rule between the lands have even influenced the way these dishes are described; certain words for foods are the same in southern Italy and Algeria. Although this salad is a popular complement to Algerian couscous, it blends well with most of the recipes in this book.

Mixed Algerian Salad

1. Preheat broiler or grill. Grill peppers until blistered (about 5–10 minutes), turning often. Remove from oven or grill, and place in paper bags for 5 minutes. Fold tops of the paper bags over, and tape them shut to enclose steam. Allow peppers to stand for 10 minutes or up to 1 hour. After the 10 minutes have passed, carefully release the steam from the paper bags. (This step can be done a day ahead of time.)

2. Peel the skin off the peppers. Cut the tops off of the peppers, and slice them into thin slices. Quarter the tomatoes. Combine peppers, tomatoes, cucumber, onions, and olives.

3. Whisk together olive oil and vinegar, and season with salt and pepper to taste. Serve at room temperature.

- 4 green bell peppers
- 4 large tomatoes
- 1 cucumber, sliced into thin rounds
- 2 small yellow onions, grated and drained, with excess liquid pressed out
- 1/4 cup black olives, pitted and sliced
- 1/4 cup extra-virgin olive oil
- 2 Tbsp vinegar
  Kosher salt, to taste
  Freshly ground pepper, to taste

Healthy Living Tradition

Tomatoes contain lots of calcium and vitamin C and are easy to grow. Even if all the land you have is a balcony, you can grow beautiful cherry tomatoes right in the pot. They make a great addition to most meals, and flash roasting them brings out their sweetness.

Exchanges/Choices			
2 Vegetable	Calories	115	Sodium 45mg
1 1/2 Fat	Calories from Fat	70	Total Carbohydrate 11g
	Total Fat	8.0g	Dietary Fiber 3g
	Saturated Fat	1.1g	Sugars 6g
Serves 8	Trans Fat	0.0g	Protein 2g
Serving Size: 1/2 cup	Cholesterol	0mg	

Vegan dish

This salad is called Shepherd's Salad because it contains feta cheese, which is normally made of a combination of sheep and goat's milk cheese. In the Mediterranean, shepherds often take a salad like this with them for lunch.

Shepherd's Salad

1. Mix tomatoes, cucumbers, bell pepper, and parsley together in a large bowl.

2. Pour lemon juice into a separate bowl, and whisk in olive oil and cumin. Pour dressing over salad, and serve with feta cheese.

4 **ripe tomatoes, diced**
1 **English or 2 Persian cucumbers, diced**
1 **green bell pepper, diced**
1 **cup fresh parsley, finely chopped**
1/4 **cup fresh lemon juice**
2 **Tbsp extra-virgin olive oil**
1/4 **tsp ground cumin**
1/4 **cup feta cheese, crumbled**

Healthy Living Tradition

This salad pairs well with many other dishes, which helps you get nutritious, healthful meals every day. Make salads a part of every meal.

Exchanges/Choices	Calories	90	Sodium	85mg
2 Vegetable	Calories from Fat	55	**Total Carbohydrate**	8g
1 Fat	**Total Fat**	6.0g	Dietary Fiber	2g
	Saturated Fat	1.6g	Sugars	4g
Serves 6	Trans Fat	0.1g	**Protein**	3g
Serving Size: 1/6 recipe	**Cholesterol**	5mg		

Originally from Lebanon, this delicious cucumber and tomato salad tossed with crunchy toasted pita pieces and dressed with pomegranate molasses will please anyone and everyone. The word *fattoush* comes from the Arabic *fattat*, which means "grown-up girl." In this sense, the salad is "grown" by the addition of leftover pita pieces. Sumac spice is obtained by grinding the seeds of the sumac plant, which is a member of the cashew family. It produces a beautiful red powder that gives a tangy taste to chicken, eggs, spice mixes, rice, and dips. The spice does not come from the poison species found in North America (such as poison ivy and poison oak).

Fattoush Salad

❈ Salata Fattoush ❈

1. Preheat broiler.

2. Combine cucumber, tomatoes, onion, and green pepper in a large salad bowl.

3. Sprinkle pita pieces with sumac, and place under broiler. Toast for 2–4 minutes, until golden on both sides. Remove pita from oven. Set aside to cool.

4. Mix olive oil, pomegranate molasses, lemon juice, salt, and pepper in a medium bowl. Whisk vigorously to form a smooth dressing.

5. Add pita chips to salad, and toss to combine. Pour dressing over salad. Toss again to combine. Serve immediately.

- 1 **cucumber, diced**
- 4 **Roma tomatoes, chopped finely**
- 1 **medium red onion, thinly sliced**
- 1 **green bell pepper, seeded and diced**
- 1 **whole-wheat pita, cut into 12 pieces**
- 1 **tsp sumac**
- 2 **Tbsp extra-virgin olive oil**
- 1 **Tbsp pomegranate molasses**
  Juice of 1 lemon (about 1/4 cup)
- 1/4 **tsp kosher salt**
- 1/4 **tsp freshly ground pepper, to taste**

Healthy Living Tradition

Toss leftover morsels of meat or chicken with this salad for a quick lunch or dinner.

Exchanges/Choices		Calories	85	Sodium	110mg
1/2 Starch • 1 Vegetable		Calories from Fat	35	Total Carbohydrate	12g
1/2 Fat		Total Fat	4.0g	Dietary Fiber	2g
		Saturated Fat	0.5g	Sugars	4g
Serves 8 / Serving Size: 1/2 cup		Trans Fat	0.0g	Protein	2g
		Cholesterol	0mg		

Vegan dish

This quick salad is a tasty and convenient way to incorporate more vegetables into your diet. It is perfect for buffets and picnics because it tastes best at room temperature.

Mixed Vegetable Salad with Tomato, Dijon, and Olive Vinaigrette

1. Place green beans, asparagus, frozen peas, and sugar snap peas in a medium saucepan. Cover with water. Bring to a boil, and reduce heat to low. Simmer for 5–10 minutes, until tender. Drain, and immediately submerge in a bowl of cold ice water. Place romaine in the bottom of a large serving bowl.

2. Preheat oven to 500°F.

3. Pour balsamic vinegar into a small bowl. Whisk in mustard until well incorporated. Whisk in olive oil until smooth. Taste, and season with salt and pepper to taste.

4. Place cherry tomatoes in a single layer on a baking sheet. Roast for 5 minutes or until charred and soft. Stir tomatoes and olives into vinaigrette. Taste dressing. If it is too sour, add sugar and stir to incorporate.

5. Drain vegetables well, and place in a salad bowl. Toss with lettuce and vinaigrette. Serve.

1	cup trimmed green beans
1	cup trimmed asparagus
1	cup frozen peas, thawed and drained
1	cup sugar snap peas, trimmed
2	cups cleaned and chopped romaine
1/4	cup balsamic vinegar
1	tsp Dijon mustard
1/4	cup extra-virgin olive oil
	Salt, to taste
	Freshly ground pepper, to taste
1/2	cup cherry tomatoes, quartered
1	Tbsp niçoise olives, pitted and chopped
1	tsp sugar, if desired

Healthy Living Tradition

Roasting or grilling tomatoes heightens their sweetness and flavor. If you find that the tomatoes you buy are not as flavorful as you'd like, try this trick. You'll have marvelous results.

Exchanges/Choices	Calories	130	Sodium	60mg
2 Vegetable	Calories from Fat	80	Total Carbohydrate	10g
2 Fat	Total Fat	9.0g	Dietary Fiber	3g
	Saturated Fat	1.3g	Sugars	4g
Serves 6	Trans Fat	0.0g	Protein	3g
Serving Size: 1/6 recipe	Cholesterol	0mg		
Vegan dish				

Adding cooked potatoes to simple salads to fortify them is a typical Sicilian touch. My great-grandmother used to slice cold boiled potatoes into her salads as part of the Sunday meal. In rural areas all over Italy, salads were often much heavier than they were in urban areas. This is due to the fact that peasants, fisherman, and shepherds alike would take salad lunches with them while they worked. Their professions required strong lunches to sustain them, but ones light enough that they would not get tired after eating them. Small amounts of eggs, potatoes, cheeses, and dried, cured meats and fish became popular additions. This trend was in contradiction of traditional multi-course meals, in which salads tend to be light, simple affairs meant to cleanse the palate before the cheese and dessert courses.

Sicilian Salad with Potatoes

1. Place potatoes in a medium saucepan, and cover with water. Bring to boil over high heat. Cook until fork-tender. Drain well, and place in a large bowl 3/4 full of cold water and ice. Let potatoes cool, drain well, and place in a large salad bowl.

2. Add cucumber, tomatoes, onion, olives, and capers. Mix to combine.

3. Pour lemon juice in a small bowl, and slowly add olive oil while whisking. Add oregano, salt, pepper, and red pepper flakes, if desired. Whisk well to combine. Pour dressing over salad, and serve.

 1 **lb golden potatoes, scrubbed, peeled, and cut into 1-inch pieces**
 1 **(12 oz) cucumber, peeled and diced**
 2 **large vine-ripened tomatoes, quartered**
 1 **small red onion, thinly sliced**
12 **black olives, pitted and halved**
 2 **Tbsp capers, rinsed and dried**
1/4 **cup freshly squeezed lemon juice**
 3 **Tbsp extra-virgin olive oil**
 1 **tsp dried oregano**
1/2 **tsp kosher salt**
1/4 **tsp freshly ground black pepper**
    Pinch red pepper flakes, if desired

Healthy Living Tradition

Olives are a great source of healthy monounsaturated fat and low in calories. They are a tasty addition to many dishes when used in moderation.

Exchanges/Choices	Calories	110	Sodium	250mg
1/2 Starch • 1 Vegetable	Calories from Fat	55	**Total Carbohydrate**	14g
1 Fat	**Total Fat**	6.0g	Dietary Fiber	2g
	Saturated Fat	0.8g	Sugars	3g
Serves 8 / **Serving Size:** 1/2 cup	Trans Fat	0.0g	**Protein**	2g
	Cholesterol	0mg		
Vegan dish				

This bright, crunchy salad is a welcome change from monotonous lettuce-based salads. Serve with *Salmon Stuffed with Spinach and Feta* (p. 122) or *Veal Scaloppine with Roasted Red Peppers and Arugula* (p. 108).

Corn, Tomato, Pea, and Dill Salad

1. Place peas in a saucepan, and cover with water. Bring to a boil over high heat, and cook for 5 minutes or until tender. Drain. Rinse with cold water.

2. Combine peas, corn, tomatoes, olive oil, dill, basil, salt, and pepper in a large bowl. Toss well to combine. Serve at room temperature.

- 1 cup sugar snap peas or English peas
- 1 cup frozen corn, thawed
- 1/2 cup cherry tomatoes, cut in half
- 2 Tbsp extra-virgin olive oil
- 1 bunch fresh baby dill, finely chopped (about 4 tbsp)
- 10 fresh basil leaves, torn
  Salt, to taste
  Freshly ground pepper, to taste

Healthy Living Tradition

Sugar snap peas contain a good amount of vitamin C. Try adding more vitamin C-rich vegetables to your diet by making unique salads like this one.

Exchanges/Choices			
1/2 Starch	**Calories**	105	
1 1/2 Fat	Calories from Fat	65	
	Total Fat	7.0g	
	Saturated Fat	1.0g	
Serves 4	Trans Fat	0.0g	
Serving Size: 1/2 cup	**Cholesterol**	0mg	

Sodium	5mg
Total Carbohydrate	10g
Dietary Fiber	2g
Sugars	2g
Protein	2g

Vegan dish

This salad's combination of fresh and cooked vegetables along with fruity olive flavor provides a great alternative to regular salads. Tapenade is an olive paste that originally hails from southern France. The name *tapenade* is said to come from the ancient Provençal word, *tapena,* which means "to cover." In this recipe, the paste replaces traditional dressing for a unique dressing. Jarred olive paste can be substituted for this homemade version. Serve this salad with grilled or roasted fish or chicken.

Cucumber, String Bean, and Olive Tapenade Salad

1. Bring a pot of water to a boil over high heat. Add string beans. Cook until tender, drain, and place beans in a bowl of cold water.

2. Split the cucumbers lengthwise. Using a spoon, remove and discard the seeds. Dice the cucumbers, and place in a large bowl.

3. Place olives, lemon juice, pepper, and olive oil in food processor, and mix to combine.

4. Add string beans to the cucumbers. Spoon olive paste over the top. Mix to combine, and serve.

1/2 cup string beans, trimmed
1 1/4 lb cucumbers
1/4 cup black olives (such as Gaeta or Kalamata), pitted
2 Tbsp freshly squeezed lemon juice
1/4 tsp freshly ground pepper
2 Tbsp extra-virgin olive oil

Healthy Living Tradition

Because conventionally grown cucumbers are normally coated with a great deal of wax, opt for organic varieties instead.

Exchanges/Choices	Calories		60	Sodium	50mg
1 Vegetable	Calories from Fat		45	Total Carbohydrate	4g
1 Fat	Total Fat		5.0g	Dietary Fiber	1g
	Saturated Fat		0.7g	Sugars	1g
Serves 6	Trans Fat		0.0g	Protein	1g
Serving Size: 1 cup	Cholesterol		0mg		

Vegan dish

Eggplant has a long and shady history in the Mediterranean region. Originally given names like "insane apple" and "demons' eggs," the eggplant is now a celebrated part of the local diet. Because this salad can be made in advance, it's great for entertaining. Try it at your next picnic.

Marinated Eggplant Salad

❋ Melintzano Salata ❋

1. Preheat broiler. Prick eggplants all over with a fork. Place eggplants on a baking sheet, and broil for 5–10 minutes or until soft. Let eggplants cool until they can be handled.

2. Meanwhile, combine tomatoes, mint, garlic, olive oil, lemon juice, salt, and pepper in a salad bowl.

3. Peel eggplants, cut off tops, and chop into bite-size pieces. Add eggplant to salad, mix well to coat, cover, and refrigerate overnight.

4. To serve, place romaine lettuce on the bottom of a serving platter. Spoon eggplant mixture on top of the lettuce.

- 3 **small eggplants (5–6 inches long)**
- 2 **medium tomatoes, chopped**
- 20 **fresh mint leaves, chopped**
- 1 **clove garlic, minced**
- 2 **Tbsp extra-virgin olive oil**
  Juice of 1 lemon
  Kosher salt, to taste
  Freshly ground pepper, to taste
- 1 **head romaine lettuce, washed, trimmed, and chopped into bite-size pieces**

Healthy Living Tradition

When buying eggplant, choose those with a bright, shiny finish without bruises. Eggplants should be slightly heavy for their size.

Exchanges/Choices			Calories	65	Sodium	10mg
2 Vegetable			Calories from Fat	30	**Total Carbohydrate**	8g
1/2 Fat			**Total Fat**	3.5g	Dietary Fiber	3g
			Saturated Fat	0.5g	Sugars	3g
Serves 8			Trans Fat	0.0g	**Protein**	1g
Serving Size: 1/2 cup			**Cholesterol**	0mg		

Vegan dish

This salad trio consists of **Zucchini Relish Salad**, **Chopped Cooked Salad**, and **Fresh Vegetable Salad**. Serving this unique combination of popular Moroccan salads makes even sensible salads seem sensuous. For dramatic effect, serve these salads on a single gold or silver charger in three separate mounds or in small Moroccan-style pottery bowls on top of a large silver or gold tray. This is the perfect way to complement a traditional North African meal.

Moroccan Salad Trio

#1. Zucchini Relish Salad

1. Place zucchini in a medium saucepan, and cover with water. Bring to a boil over high heat, reduce heat to low, and simmer for 10–15 minutes or until zucchini is fork-tender. Place zucchini in a medium bowl and mash them. Mix in lemon juice, salt, garlic, hot sauce, caraway seeds, red pepper flakes. Mix well and refrigerate. To serve: taste, and adjust seasoning if necessary, top with olive oil.

- 2 medium zucchini, trimmed and quartered
- Juice of 1/2 lemon
- 1/4 tsp kosher salt
- 1 clove garlic, minced
- Dash Moroccan harissa or other hot sauce
- 1/2 tsp caraway seeds
- Dash crushed red pepper flakes
- 1 tsp extra-virgin olive oil

Zucchini Relish Salad - Exchanges/Choices	Calories	20	Sodium	85mg
1 Vegetable	Calories from Fat	10	Total Carbohydrate	3g
	Total Fat	1.0g	Dietary Fiber	1g
Serves 6 • Serving Size: 1/6 recipe	Saturated Fat	0.1g	Sugars	1g
	Trans Fat	0.0g	Protein	1g
Vegan dish	Cholesterol	0mg		

Healthy Living Tradition

North Africans often serve numerous salads to accompany the main course of couscous and tajines. By serving more than one salad at a time, you'll increase your fiber and nutrient intake and fill up on healthy vegetables instead of carbohydrates and proteins alone.

Moroccan Salad Trio Exchanges/Choices	Calories	300	Sodium	155mg
4 Vegetable • 4 1/2 Fat	Calories from Fat	205	Total Carbohydrate	25g
	Total Fat	23.0g	Dietary Fiber	6g
Serves 6 / Serving Size: 1/6 recipe	Saturated Fat	3.0g	Sugars	12g
	Trans Fat	0.0g	Protein	5g
Vegan dish	Cholesterol	0mg		

#2. Chopped Cooked Salad

1. Place the tomatoes, onion, cucumber, and green bell pepper in a saucepan. Add water to cover, and bring to a boil over high heat. Reduce heat to low, and simmer, uncovered, for 5 minutes. Allow to cool.

2. In a small bowl, combine lemon juice, olive oil, and garlic.

3. Strain the vegetables, and place in a bowl. Stir in dressing and cilantro. Season with salt and pepper to taste.

2 **large tomatoes, quartered**
1 **yellow onion, finely chopped**
1/2 **cucumber, seeded and sliced**
1 **green bell pepper, diced**
Juice of 1 lemon
3 **Tbsp extra-virgin olive oil**
2 **cloves garlic, minced**
2 **Tbsp fresh cilantro, finely chopped**
Kosher salt, to taste
Freshly ground pepper, to taste

Chopped Cooked Salad	Calories	90	Sodium	5mg
Exchanges/Choices	Calories from Fat	65	**Total Carbohydrate**	8g
1 Vegetable	**Total Fat**	7.0g	Dietary Fiber	2g
1 Fat	Saturated Fat	1.0g	Sugars	4g
	Trans Fat	0.0g	**Protein**	1g
Serves 6 / **Serving Size:** 1/6 recipe	**Cholesterol**	0mg		

Vegan dish

#3. Fresh Vegetable Salad

1. Heat 1 Tbsp olive oil in a small skillet over low heat. Add almonds. Cook, stirring occasionally, until lightly golden. Be careful not to burn the almonds.

2. In a large bowl, combine tomatoes, cucumbers, bell peppers, radishes, olives, onion, and corn.

3. In a small bowl, whisk together lemon juice and remaining 1/4 cup olive oil. Add salt and pepper to taste. Combine dressing with vegetables, and mix well to coat. Sprinkle almonds on top of salad before serving.

1/4 **cup + 1 Tbsp extra-virgin olive oil, divided**
1/4 **cup blanched slivered almonds**
3 **Roma tomatoes, diced**
3 **Persian cucumbers or 1 English cucumber, diced**
1 **green bell pepper, diced**
2 **red bell peppers, diced**
6 **radishes, grated**
1/4 **cup green or black olives, pitted and sliced**
1 **yellow onion, grated**
1/2 **cup frozen corn, thawed and drained**
1/2 **cup lemon juice**
Kosher salt, to taste
Freshly ground pepper, to taste

Fresh Vegetable Salad	Calories	190	Sodium	60mg
Exchanges/Choices	Calories from Fat	135	**Total Carbohydrate**	15g
3 Vegetable	**Total Fat**	15.0g	Dietary Fiber	4g
2 1/2 Fat	Saturated Fat	1.9g	Sugars	7g
	Trans Fat	0.0g	**Protein**	3g
Serves 6 / **Serving Size:** 1/6 recipe	**Cholesterol**	0mg		

Vegan dish

This is one of my all-time favorite Italian salads. It's simple and nutritious. It's also a great lunch-time salad for busy days at the office.

Mozzarella, Tomato, and Chickpea Salad

1. Combine mozzarella balls, tomatoes, and chickpeas in a medium bowl. Add olive oil. Stir, taste, and add salt and pepper to taste.

2. Wash spinach, and layer it in the bottom of a serving bowl. Arrange mozzarella-tomato-chickpea mixture on top of spinach. Serve at room temperature.

2.5 oz fresh mozzarella balls, drained
1 cup cherry tomatoes
1 cup no-salt-added canned chickpeas
2 tsp extra-virgin olive oil
Kosher salt, to taste
Freshly ground pepper, to taste
12 oz fresh baby spinach

Healthy Living Tradition

To make a meal out of this salad, add leftover shredded turkey or chicken and croutons. Spinach contains tons of iron, calcium, and vitamins. It is not only tasty, but a healthful ingredient in dishes across the Mediterranean as well.

Exchanges/Choices			
1/2 Starch	Calories	155	Sodium 165mg
1 Vegetable	Calories from Fat	65	Total Carbohydrate 16g
1 Lean Meat	Total Fat	7.0g	Dietary Fiber 5g
1 Fat	Saturated Fat	2.3g	Sugars 4g
	Trans Fat	0.0g	Protein 10g
	Cholesterol	5mg	

Serves 4
Serving Size: 1/2 cup

I like to make this salad at New Year's because it combines lentils, which are representative of wealth and fortune; pomegranate seeds, which represent passion and vitality; and crisp greens, which are representative of healthfulness. By serving this dish to guests, you're offering them good tidings of wealth, love, health, and longevity all in one. In addition, the contrasting red, green, and brown colors are stunning, and the crunch of the pomegranate seeds is the perfect contrast to the tender lentils.

New Year's Lentil Salad

1. Place lentils in a medium saucepan, and cover with water. Bring to a boil over high heat, reduce heat to low, and add bay leaf. Simmer, uncovered, for 30 minutes or until tender. Drain, discard bay leaf, and reserve.

2. Divide mixed greens evenly among four salad plates. Sprinkle pomegranate seeds over the lettuce.

3. In a small bowl, whisk together pomegranate juice and molasses. Slowly pour in olive oil while whisking vigorously to form a homogenous dressing. Season with salt and pepper to taste. Sprinkle lentils evenly over salad. Drizzle dressing over the top.

1/2 cup lentils, rinsed, drained, and sorted
1 bay leaf
4 cups mixed field greens or baby greens
1 ripe pomegranate, seeds removed and juice reserved (about 1/2 cup seeds and 1/2 cup juice)
1 tsp pomegranate molasses
2 Tbsp extra-virgin olive oil
Salt, to taste
Freshly ground pepper, to taste

Healthy Living Tradition

Throughout history, pomegranate juice and seeds were used in natural medicines to cure a wide variety of ailments. They are now grown in California and Arizona.

Exchanges/Choices	Calories	185	Sodium	15mg
1 Starch	Calories from Fat	65	**Total Carbohydrate**	24g
1/2 Fruit	**Total Fat**	7.0g	Dietary Fiber	7g
1 Lean Meat	Saturated Fat	1.0g	Sugars	10g
1 Fat	Trans Fat	0.0g	**Protein**	7g
	Cholesterol	0mg		

Serves 4
Serving Size: 1 1/4 cups

Vegan dish

Fantastic Finales

Desserts in the Mediterranean range from humble concoctions made out of fruit and healthful ingredients to elegant and elaborate creations that are as deliciously complex to look at as they are to eat. The simple, straightforward types of desserts are prepared in homes, whereas the intricate recipes are usually purchased from pastry shops. Because they are richer and more fattening, the pastry-shop desserts are usually reserved for special occasions. This chapter contains home-style Mediterranean desserts, which are meant to provide a sweet end to a healthful homemade meal anytime.

Historically, it is important to note that not all of the countries in the region had sugar until relatively recently. The ancient Egyptians obtained sugar from the Persians. Pictures from Ramses II's tomb depict bakeries where sugar-filled treats were prepared for royalty. Cleopatra was also known for her love of sugar. Commoners, meanwhile, had to make do with molasses and honey. It wasn't until the 18th century in France that sugar became widely available for culinary purposes. Originally it was very expensive and sold in apothecary shops as a medicine. The expensive price of sugar made it unavailable for many, and fruit was often eaten at the end of a meal. While our modern palates have changed, sometimes the old ways are best. Eating a piece of fruit instead of a sugar- and fat-laden dessert is a better choice for everyone. When the occasion calls for something extra, however, the following recipes will allow you to enjoy dessert with both pleasure and health in mind.

The desserts featured in this chapter were originally developed to showcase seasonal bounty and utilize household staples. I purposely selected these recipes because they are sweet and luscious, yet healthful. They contain no artificial sweeteners. By adopting a Mediterranean philosophy in our own kitchens, we can make desserts that are simple, tasty, and satisfying for all of life's occasions.

You'll sample Italian cookies, like *Anise Biscuits* (p. 195), *Calabrian Sesame Cookies* (p. 198), and *Tuscan Cantucci Cookies* (p. 199), which have been made in the same manner for centuries. These cookies are more than just a quick treat; they are links to the land from which they come. Certain family gatherings and celebrations would not be the same without them. They make great edible gifts as well. For a more substantial Italian dessert, try *Italian Sponge Cake* (p. 202), *Pineapple Tiramisu* (p. 203), or *Strawberry Mascarpone Parfaits* (p. 204). They will soon become family favorites.

If you're in the mood for a pudding, *Baked Egyptian Pumpkin Pudding* (p. 205), *Lemony Rice Pudding* (p. 206), *Milk and Rose Water Pudding* (p. 207), *Sweet Couscous* (p. 208), and *Yogurt Custard with Figs and Pistachios* (p. 210) are sweet and comforting. These puddings have been traditionally popular in the Middle East, where they are a perfect finale to a homemade meal with family and friends. In addition to the Middle Eastern puddings, you will find recipes in which phyllo dough is used to encase fresh and dried fruit, such as the *Apple, Date, and Raisin Phyllo Strudel* (p. 212) and the *Fruit-Filled Phyllo Snake* (p. 214).

During hot weather, the Italian flavored ices, such as the *Espresso Granita* (p. 217), *Watermelon and Rose Water Granita* (p. 218), and *Raspberry and Lemon Sorbet* (p. 219), can't be beat. Traditional Moroccan tangerines take center stage in the *Moroccan Tangerine Sorbet* (p. 220). Typical French desserts, like *French Meringue with Rose Cream* (p. 221), *Grapes with Goat Cheese and Almonds* (p. 222), and *Melon, Plum, and Nectarine Soup* (p. 224), are all very refreshing in the summer months. In addition, *Nectarines with Mint Sugar* (p. 225), *Peaches in Basil-Yogurt Cream* (p. 226), *Poached Apples in Rose Tea* (p. 227), *Sweet Fried Plantains* (p. 228), and *Fresh Figs with Raspberry Purée* (p. 229) prove that fresh ingredients and a simple application are all that is needed to produce extraordinary tastes.

These crunchy cookies were first introduced in the U.S. by Italian immigrants. Italians had enjoyed these cookies since ancient times, when the Romans would take them on long voyages because they stayed fresh for a long time. These cookies are also very popular in the northern coastal areas of Egypt. Because the ancient Romans were attracted to Egypt for its large granaries and the ancient Egyptians already possessed sugar and sophisticated bakeries, it is likely that the Romans learned the recipe from their stay in Egypt. Enjoy this recipe with *Classic Italian Espresso* (p. 247).

Anise Biscuits

❈ *Biscotti d'Anice* ❈

1. Preheat the oven to 375°F. Grease and flour two (8 1/2 × 4 1/2 × 2 1/2-inch) loaf pans.

2. In a large bowl, add eggs, and whisk by hand or with an electric mixer on high speed until the mixture turns light yellow, about 3 minutes. Slowly add the sugar, and continue to beat until incorporated. With the mixer running on low speed, add the flour, anise seeds, and vanilla. Mix well to incorporate. Pour half of the batter into each pan. Smooth out the top of the batter.

3. Bake in the middle of the oven for 25 minutes or until dough turns golden. Remove from the oven. Reduce temperature to 325°F. Let biscotti cool for 10 minutes in the pan. Using oven mitts, turn over loaf pans to unmold cookies. Let cool for 10 minutes.

4. Cut each loaf crosswise into 1-inch sections. Lay each slice on its side on a cookie sheet. Bake for 8–10 minutes, remove from oven, turn biscotti over, and bake for another 8–10 minutes. Cookies should be light brown when finished. Cool thoroughly. Cookies will keep in an airtight container for up to a month.

4	large eggs, at room temperature
3/4	cup sugar
2	cups unbleached, all-purpose flour
2	tsp anise seeds
1	tsp vanilla or anise extract

Healthy Living Tradition

Keep light dessert recipes like this one on hand to satisfy sweet cravings without going overboard with calories and fat.

Exchanges/Choices		Calories	150	Sodium	25mg
2 Carbohydrate		Calories from Fat	20	**Total Carbohydrate**	29g
		Total Fat	2.0g	Dietary Fiber	1g
Serves 12		Saturated Fat	0.6g	Sugars	13g
Serving Size: 2		Trans Fat	0.0g	**Protein**	4g
		Cholesterol	70mg		

Amaretti **are the light, airy, and wonderfully chewy almond macaroons from Italy.** The Lazzaroni company of Saronno produces tins full of this wonderful treat, each containing pretty little paper packets with two *amaretti* back to back. According to legend, the recipe dates from 1718 and honors the Cardinal of Milan's visit to the town of Saronno (which was under the municipality of Milan). A young couple thought of the recipe, and the idea of wrapping two cookies together to symbolize their love. Enchanted with the idea, the Cardinal blessed them and married them, and they lived happily ever after. The original recipe contains cherry kernels instead of almond extract, and its precise details are a tightly guarded secret. *Amaretti di Saronno* are also crushed and used in Italian desserts the way gingersnaps and Oreos are used in American desserts. Here is my version, which I make for friends and family.

Almond Macaroons

❋ *Amaretti* ❋

1. Grind half of the almonds to dust in a food processor. Transfer ground almonds to a bowl.

2. Grind the rest of the almonds to dust, and transfer to the bowl. Add sugar and extracts. Mix well, and set aside.

3. Place egg whites in a bowl fitted to a standing electric mixer fitted with the whisk attachment. Whisk egg whites on low speed, and gradually increase the speed to high. Add salt. Beat for 5 minutes or until whites are stiff.

1 1/2 cups blanched almonds
1/2 cup sugar
2 tsp almond extract
1 tsp vanilla extract
2 egg whites
1/8 tsp salt

4. With a rubber spatula, gradually fold nut mixture into egg-white mixture as gently as possible until fully incorporated (no egg white is showing).

5. Line two cookie sheets with parchment paper or silicone mats. Spoon teaspoonfuls of mixture about 1 1/2 inches apart on cookie sheets. Let stand for 15 minutes, and preheat the oven to 300°F. Bake on the center rack of the oven for 15–20 minutes or until light golden. Cool cookies on a wire rack, and store in an airtight container for up to a month.

Healthy Living Tradition

Ground almonds produce almond flour, a common ingredient in the Mediterranean. In addition to its wonderful taste, ground almonds give character to pie and torte crusts and can be substituted for regular flour in many recipes.

Exchanges/Choices		Calories	115	Sodium	30mg
1/2 Carbohydrate		Calories from Fat	65	**Total Carbohydrate**	10g
1 1/2 Fat		**Total Fat**	7.0g	Dietary Fiber	2g
		Saturated Fat	0.6g	Sugars	8g
Serves 15		Trans Fat	0.0g	**Protein**	4g
Serving Size: 2 cookies		**Cholesterol**	0mg		

These are called "Queen's Cookies" in Italy. In the southern Italian province of Calabria, these cookies are served on Christmas day (to honor Jesus being born unto the Virgin Mary) and at weddings. These simple-to-make cookies can be made a month ahead of time and frozen.

Calabrian Sesame Cookies

❋ Biscotti di Regina ❋

1. Preheat oven to 375°F. Line two cookie sheets with parchment paper or silicone liners.

2. Combine flour, sugar, baking powder, and salt in a large bowl. Stir in canola oil, and mix well to combine. Combine milk and vanilla in a small bowl, and stir into mixture. Mix ingredients well to form a dough, and turn out onto a lightly floured work surface.

3. Pour sesame seeds onto a plate. Break off 1-inch pieces of dough, and roll them to create finger shapes. Roll in sesame seeds to coat. Place on baking sheets, and slightly flatten top of cookies with a finger. Bake for 18–20 minutes or until very light gold in color.

2 1/4 cups unbleached all-purpose flour, plus extra for work surface
1/3 cup sugar
1 1/2 tsp baking powder
   Pinch salt
1/4 cup canola oil, placed in freezer for 20 minutes before using
1/4 cup 1% milk
2 tsp vanilla extract
3/4 cup sesame seeds, untoasted

Healthy Living Tradition

Sweets (especially those relatively low in sugar, like this one) can be part of a healthy lifestyle. If you are planning on eating dessert after a meal, make sure to account for that extra carbohydrate when you decide what to eat for dinner.

Exchanges/Choices		Calories	160	Sodium	40mg
1 1/2 Carbohydrate		Calories from Fat	65	**Total Carbohydrate**	21g
1 1/2 Fat		**Total Fat**	7.0g	Dietary Fiber	1g
		Saturated Fat	0.8g	Sugars	5g
Serves 15		Trans Fat	0.0g	**Protein**	3g
Serving Size: 2 cookies		**Cholesterol**	0mg		

In the dreamy Tuscan hillside town of Chiusure, *cantucci* are served at breakfast, for dessert, and as snacks. These crunchy honey- and lemon-flavored biscotti are simple to make and a joy to eat. If you've never made biscotti before, don't be intimidated! In the ancient world, this type of cookie was packed onto trade ships. Because of their crisp, twice-baked exterior, they last for weeks.

Tuscan Cantucci Cookies

❋ Cantucci ❋

1. Preheat oven to 375°F. Line a large baking sheet with parchment paper or silicone mats.

2. Stir flour, 3/4 cup sugar, baking powder, and salt in a large bowl to combine.

3. In a separate bowl, combine eggs, honey, lemon juice, lemon zest, vanilla extract, and almond extract. Mix well. Pour egg mixture into flour mixture, and stir until incorporated. Stir in almonds. Drop dough onto baking sheet to make two 14 × 4-inch logs that are spaced 2–3 inches apart. Wet your fingertips, and smooth out the logs to even shapes. Sprinkle logs with 1 Tbsp sugar. Bake for 20–25 minutes or until logs are golden. Remove logs from oven, and let cool on the baking sheet for 10 minutes.

4. Reduce oven temperature to 325°F. Locate a clean baking sheet. Carefully transfer logs to work surface and, using a serrated knife, cut them into 1/2-inch-thick slices. Arrange slices on their sides on the clean baking sheet. Bake for about 10 minutes or until cantucci are golden. Cool completely. Store in an airtight container. Serve with espresso, cappuccino, or caffé latte for dunking.

- 2 1/4 cups unbleached, all-purpose flour
- 3/4 cup + 1 Tbsp sugar, divided
- 2 tsp baking powder
- 3/4 tsp salt
- 4 large eggs
- 2 Tbsp honey
- 2 Tbsp lemon juice
- 1 Tbsp lemon zest
- 2 tsp vanilla extract
- 1 tsp almond extract
- 1 cup blanched whole almonds, toasted

Healthy Living Tradition

Giving homemade gifts feels great! Why not give half of these cookies as a gift? The recipient will be delighted.

Exchanges/Choices				
1 Starch	Calories	105	Sodium	100mg
1/2 Fat	Calories from Fat	30	Total Carbohydrate	16g
	Total Fat	3.5g	Dietary Fiber	1g
Serves 28	Saturated Fat	0.4g	Sugars	8g
	Trans Fat	0.0g	Protein	3g
Serving Size: 1 cookie	Cholesterol	30mg		

Crostate are Italian pies that can be filled with everything from preserves to fresh fruit and chocolate. They tend to be less sugary than American pies. The crust in this version uses oil. If you prefer to use butter for a traditional crust, substitute 1/2 cup (1 stick) unsalted butter at room temperature for the oil listed in the ingredients. Frozen berries also work well in this recipe. You can also use a 10-inch pan with a removable bottom to make a large crostata instead of mini ones.

Mini Mixed Berry Crostata

1. In a food processor fitted with a metal blade, combine flour and oil until crumbly. Add egg, 2 Tbsp sugar, and water. Mix dough until it is completely softened and begins to form a ball. Place on plastic wrap, and work into a ball. Cover with plastic wrap, and refrigerate 1 hour.

2. Prepare the filling by combining strawberries, blackberries, raspberries, and blueberries in a medium saucepan. Add cornstarch mixture, cinnamon stick, and 1/3 cup sugar. Bring to a boil over high heat, reduce heat to medium, stir slowly, and continue to cook for 3–5 minutes, until mixture becomes thick like a pie filling. Remove from heat, and let cool. Discard cinnamon stick.

2 1/2 cups unbleached, all-purpose flour
1/3 cup vegetable or canola oil, placed in a jar in the freezer for 45 minutes
1 egg
2 Tbsp + 1/3 cup sugar, divided
4–6 Tbsp water
1/4 cup trimmed strawberries
1/4 cup blackberries
1/4 cup raspberries
1/4 cup blueberries
3 tsp cornstarch, in 1/4 cup water
1 cinnamon stick
   Nonstick cooking spray
1 egg white, lightly beaten
10 fresh mint leaves

3. When dough has been chilled, preheat oven to 400°F. Spray five (4-inch) tart pans with nonstick cooking spray. Roll dough out into a 12-inch circle. Use the mini tart pans as cookie cutters to cut out 10 circles in the dough (scraping up and re-rolling extra dough, if necessary). Press dough down into tart shells, and prick with a fork. Line with foil. Fill with pie weights, rice, or dried beans to help pie crusts maintain their shape. Bake for 20 minutes.

4. Remove from oven. Remove foil, discard rice or beans, and brush with egg white. Return crusts to oven. Bake another 10 minutes. Let cool slightly, and carefully remove crusts from the pans. Fill each one with berry filling, and top with a mint sprig.

Healthy Living Tradition

Keep this crust recipe on hand, and use it when you crave the texture of pie, but don't want all of the excess fat and calories. You can never go wrong by using fresh, seasonal fruit as a filling.

Exchanges/Choices			
2 1/2 Carbohydrate	Calories	230	Sodium 15mg
1 1/2 Fat	Calories from Fat	70	Total Carbohydrate 35g
	Total Fat	8.0g	Dietary Fiber 1g
	Saturated Fat	0.7g	Sugars 11g
Serves 10	Trans Fat	0.0g	**Protein** 4g
Serving Size: 1 mini crostata	**Cholesterol**	20mg	

This classic Italian cake, called "Spanish Bread," can be eaten for breakfast or as a snack or used as a base for more elaborate holiday desserts. It's also a delicious base for shortcakes and sundaes. You can double the recipe, and freeze one cake after wrapping it in plastic wrap.

Italian Sponge Cake

❋ *Pan di Spagna* ❋

1. Preheat oven to 350°F. Grease a 1 1/2-quart (8.25 × 9 × 2.75-inch) loaf pan with nonstick cooking spray.

2. Beat egg whites in a large bowl until stiff. Set aside.

3. Cream sugar and egg yolks together, and continue beating until they are very light yellow in color. Stir in the vanilla. Gently fold the egg whites into the batter. Sprinkle flour on top of mixture, and carefully incorporate into the batter until just combined. Pour into prepared loaf pan, and bake for 40 minutes or until cake is golden and sides begin to pull away from the pan. Remove from the oven, and let cool completely.

Nonstick cooking spray
6 **large egg whites**
1 **cup sugar**
6 **large egg yolks**
2 **tsp vanilla**
1 1/8 **cup unbleached all-purpose flour**

Healthy Living Tradition

Adopt a healthy Italian attitude when it comes to dessert consumption. Many home-style Italian desserts are less sweet than their American counterparts. They are served to showcase seasonal fruit and are only present at celebratory meals and special occasions. By serving desserts with less sugar and fat—and eating them less often—you will be able to better control your blood glucose levels.

Exchanges/Choices		Calories	175	Sodium	35mg
2 Carbohydrate		Calories from Fat	25	**Total Carbohydrate**	31g
1/2 Fat		**Total Fat**	3.0g	Dietary Fiber	0g
		Saturated Fat	1.2g	Sugars	21g
Serves 10		Trans Fat	0.0g	**Protein**	5g
Serving Size: 1 slice		**Cholesterol**	130mg		

The rich, indulgent flavors of traditional tiramisu are reserved for special occasions in Italy. This version combines yogurt and pineapple for a light, uplifting version that is perfect for a healthy indulgence any time of year. Keep in mind that the tiramisu needs to set for a minimum of 1 hour or overnight. Diced, canned peaches or apricots can also be used in this easy recipe.

Pineapple Tiramisu

❀ *Tiramisu d'Ananas* ❀

1. Line the bottom of an 8-inch-wide bowl with 12 ladyfingers (you may need to break a few to get them to fit into holes), making an even layer. Pour or spoon half of the reserved pineapple juice over the ladyfingers.

2. Combine yogurt with cinnamon in a medium bowl. Evenly spoon yogurt mixture over ladyfingers. Scatter crushed pineapple over the yogurt, reserving 1 Tbsp for garnish. Line the top of the pineapple with remaining 12 ladyfingers. Pour remaining pineapple juice over the ladyfingers.

3. Place cocoa powder in a small sieve. Sift over the top of the ladyfingers. Place remaining 1 Tbsp crushed pineapple in the center of the tiramisu. Refrigerate for 1 hour or overnight. Divide tiramisu into eight small dessert cups, and garnish each with a mint sprig.

1 (7-oz) package (24 total) ladyfingers
1 (20-oz) can crushed pineapple with juice, juice drained and reserved
2 cups organic low-fat vanilla yogurt
1 tsp cinnamon
1 tsp natural unsweetened cocoa powder
8 fresh mint sprigs

Healthy Living Tradition

Pineapples are rich in vitamin C and manganese. To get these wonderful nutrients, try adding more pineapple to your meal plan.

Exchanges/Choices				
2 1/2 Carbohydrate	Calories	180	Sodium	75mg
	Calories from Fat	20	Total Carbohydrate	38g
	Total Fat	2.5g	Dietary Fiber	1g
Serves 8	Saturated Fat	1.0g	Sugars	27g
Serving Size: 1/2 cup	Trans Fat	0.0g	Protein	5g
	Cholesterol	30mg		

Mascarpone is a soft Italian cream cheese. It is so creamy and smooth that only a small bit of it is needed to add depth and character to an otherwise ordinary recipe. This dessert is so delicious that no one will ever suspect that it's healthy, and it can be made in only a few minutes. Save this recipe for spring and summer, when strawberries are at their peak.

Strawberry Mascarpone Parfaits

1. Place a colander in a bowl. Add yogurt. Set in the refrigerator for 6 hours or overnight.

2. Place 1 cup strawberries, mascarpone, sugar, and cinnamon in a blender, and whip until light. Stir in yogurt. Pour 1/3 cup of mixture into each of 6 clear parfait glasses. Top with 1 layer of remaining strawberry slices (reserving 6 for garnish). Scatter 1 Tbsp granola on top of the strawberry slices in each glass. Top each glass with another layer of remaining strawberry mixture. Add another layer of 1 Tbsp granola on top of the strawberry mixture in each glass. Garnish each glass with 1 remaining strawberry slice. Cover with plastic wrap, and refrigerate for at least 2 hours to a maximum of overnight before serving.

1	cup low-fat vanilla yogurt, drained
1 1/2	cups trimmed strawberries, thinly sliced
3/4	oz mascarpone
1	Tbsp sugar
1	tsp cinnamon
3/4	cup (12 Tbsp) low-fat almond granola

Healthy Living Tradition

Freeze this strawberry mixture in Popsicle molds for a healthier summertime alternative to ice cream.

Exchanges/Choices	Calories	115	Sodium	20mg
1 1/2 Carbohydrate	Calories from Fat	25	**Total Carbohydrate**	20g
1/2 Fat	**Total Fat**	3.0g	Dietary Fiber	2g
	Saturated Fat	1.4g	Sugars	12g
Serves 6	Trans Fat	0.1g	**Protein**	3g
Serving Size: 3/4 cup	**Cholesterol**	5mg		

If you love pumpkin pie filling, but always leave the crust, this is the dessert for you. It's my version of a traditional country Egyptian dessert made during the pumpkin harvest. This recipe can be put together in a few minutes and bakes quickly. Best of all, it reminds everyone of holidays, home, and family, regardless of the time of year when it's eaten. The pudding can also be made and served in individual ramekins.

Baked Egyptian Pumpkin Pudding
✻ Mahallibayat Ar Asali Fee al Forn ✻

1. Preheat oven to 350°F. Grease a 9-inch pie dish or other baking dish with nonstick cooking spray.

2. Mix together pumpkin purée, sugar, egg, cinnamon, cardamom, cloves, and raisins. Pour into prepared baking dish, and smooth out the top. Sprinkle almonds in a single layer over the top. Bake for 20 minutes or until almonds are slightly golden. Remove from oven, and let cool slightly. Divide pudding into six small bowls. Top each with 1 tsp vanilla yogurt, if desired. Sprinkle cinnamon on top, and serve.

Nonstick cooking spray
1 (15-oz) can pumpkin purée
1/3 cup sugar
1 large egg
1 tsp ground cinnamon, plus extra for sprinkling as a garnish
1/2 tsp ground cardamom
1/2 tsp ground cloves
1/4 cup raisins
1/4 cup sliced almonds
6 tsp low-fat vanilla yogurt, optional, for serving

Healthy Living Tradition

Pumpkins contain a ton of vitamin A. To get more of this in your diet, look overseas. Pumpkins are popular in many international cuisines and can be prepared in either sweet or savory dishes.

Exchanges/Choices	Calories	120	Sodium	15mg
1 1/2 Carbohydrate	Calories from Fat	25	Total Carbohydrate	23g
1/2 Fat	Total Fat	3.0g	Dietary Fiber	3g
	Saturated Fat	0.5g	Sugars	17g
Serves 6	Trans Fat	0.0g	Protein	3g
Serving Size: 1/2 cup	Cholesterol	35mg		

Many versions of sweet, citrusy, and creamy rice puddings are common in the Mediterranean. Housewives love them because they require hardly any effort, and everyone else loves their mellow, comforting flavor.

Lemony Rice Pudding

1. Rinse rice. Drain well. Pour milk into a medium saucepan. Add drained rice, cinnamon stick, lemon peel, lemon juice, and sugar. Stir with a wooden spoon, and bring to a boil over medium-high heat. Once mixture boils, reduce heat to low, stir, and cover. Simmer for 3 hours, stirring occasionally, until rice is tender and liquid is absorbed. Remove and discard cinnamon stick. Allow pudding to cool at room temperature. Pour into a serving bowl. Refrigerate leftovers for up to 2 days.

1/3	cup Egyptian, Arborio, or short-grain rice, uncooked
3 1/4	cups nonfat milk
1	cinnamon stick
	Grated peel of 1 lemon
1/4	cup freshly squeezed lemon juice
2/3	cup sugar

Healthy Living Tradition

The essential oils from citrus peel and deep notes of spices add complexity, taste, and richness to recipes without adding sugar and calories. Try cutting down on some of the sugar content in your favorite dessert recipes by adding interesting citrus and spice combinations. Cinnamon and lemon, orange and cardamom, and lime and ginger are perfect partners.

Exchanges/Choices	Calories	130	Sodium	55mg
2 Carbohydrate	Calories from Fat	0	**Total Carbohydrate**	28g
	Total Fat	0.0g	Dietary Fiber	0g
Serves 8	Saturated Fat	0.1g	Sugars	22g
Serving Size: 1/2 cup	Trans Fat	0.0g	**Protein**	4g
	Cholesterol	0mg		

Mahallibeya **is a smooth and creamy pudding traditionally made with rice flour.** It is usually served alone and is a Middle Eastern classic. Do not use a metal whisk to prepare this recipe because the metal will cause the pudding to separate.

Milk and Rose Water Pudding

�֎ Mahallibeya �֎

1. Pour milk into a medium saucepan. Add sugar and rose water. Heat, uncovered, over medium heat until boiling, stirring constantly.

2. Mix cornstarch with 1/4 cup water. Slowly add cornstarch mixture to the saucepan. Whisk vigorously. Boil pudding for 2 minutes, stirring, and reduce heat to low. Continue stirring with a wooden spoon, and cook until thick, 15–20 minutes. When the pudding has reduced to at least half of its original volume, set it aside to cool.

3. After it has cooled, pour the pudding into individual custard bowls. Refrigerate until pudding sets. To serve, garnish with ground almonds.

2 1/2	**cups 1% milk**
1/3	**cup sugar**
1	**tsp rose water**
3 1/2	**Tbsp cornstarch**
1/4	**cup ground almonds, blanched**

Healthy Living Tradition

Light, refreshing desserts like this one add the perfect sweet finish to a meal. Keep this one on hand for the kids, who will love it as well.

Exchanges/Choices					
1/2 Fat-Free Milk	**Calories**	200	**Sodium**	70mg	
1 1/2 Carbohydrate	Calories from Fat	55	**Total Carbohydrate**	32g	
1 Fat	**Total Fat**	6.0g	Dietary Fiber	1g	
	Saturated Fat	1.3g	Sugars	25g	
	Trans Fat	0.0g	**Protein**	7g	
Serves 4	**Cholesterol**	10mg			
Serving Size: 1/2 cup					

Couscous-based desserts are popular in Morocco, Tunisia, Algeria, and the Italian province of Sicily. The Sicilians inherited the couscous recipes from years of Arab rule and now enjoy savory couscous recipes, as well as sweet versions like this one. This dessert is actually a Sicilian fusion of two widely popular Arabic desserts—a traditional couscous pudding and a milk pudding known as *Mahallibeya*. By combining both recipes, this dessert has a sweet and creamy, yet crunchy and nutty consistency. Keep in mind that this dessert should be chilled completely (for at least 5 hours) before serving. It can be made a day ahead of time and holds up well in the refrigerator.

Sweet Couscous

❋ *Cuscus Dolce* ❋

1. Preheat oven to 375°F. Bring 1/2 cup milk to a boil over high heat. Turn off heat, and stir in the couscous, 1 Tbsp sugar, and salt. Cover, and let stand for 10 minutes.

2. Meanwhile, place the almonds on a cookie sheet, and toast for 5–10 minutes, until slightly golden. Let cool, and place in a food processor. Process until finely ground.

3. Remove the lid from the couscous, fluff with a fork, and stir in the almonds. Spoon mixture into a 9-inch glass or ceramic baking dish.

2 1/2 cups nonfat milk, divided
2/3 cup couscous
1/2 cup + 1 Tbsp sugar, divided
1/8 tsp salt
1 cup blanched whole almonds
4 Tbsp cornstarch, dissolved in 1/4 cup nonfat milk
1/2 cup raw unsalted pistachios, shelled and ground, or blanched almonds
1 tsp cinnamon, for topping

4. In a small bowl, combine the cornstarch with 1/4 cup milk.

5. In a medium saucepan, combine cornstarch-milk mixture, remaining 1 3/4 cups milk, and sugar over medium heat. Stir slowly and constantly with a wooden spoon in the same direction, being sure to scrape down the sides and bottom of the pan with each stir. Cook mixture until it thickens (about 20 minutes). Pudding is done when it coats the back of a spoon and its volume has been reduced by about half. Stir pistachios into the pudding. Spread pudding on top of the couscous. Sprinkle with cinnamon. Let cool, cover with plastic wrap, and refrigerate for 5 hours or until chilled.

Healthy Living Tradition

Nut- and grain-based desserts are healthy indulgences for special occasions and when eaten in moderation. Try substituting them for less healthy desserts.

Exchanges/Choices	Calories	185	Sodium	55mg
1 1/2 Carbohydrate	Calories from Fat	65	**Total Carbohydrate**	25g
1 1/2 Fat	**Total Fat**	7.0g	Dietary Fiber	2g
	Saturated Fat	0.6g	Sugars	13g
Serves 12	Trans Fat	0.0g	**Protein**	6g
Serving Size: 1/2 cup	**Cholesterol**	0mg		

Yogurt and fresh figs is an extraordinarily sweet and creamy combination that starts the days of many people in eastern Mediterranean countries, like Greece and Turkey. In this recipe, I've made a custard out of the yogurt, so you can end your day with this delightful dish.

Yogurt Custard with Figs and Pistachios

1. Combine yogurt, vanilla, almond, cornstarch mixture, cinnamon, agave nectar, and orange blossom water in a medium saucepan. Bring mixture to boil over medium-high heat while stirring slowly, but constantly, with a wooden spoon. Allow mixture to boil for 2 minutes, reduce heat to low, and stir slowly for 10 minutes or until mixture has thickened and coats the back of a spoon. Take mixture off of flame. Cover the top of the actual custard with wax paper to prevent a skin from forming. When custard is cool, spoon it into small dessert bowls or cups. Garnish each with a sprinkling of pistachios and a fig.

- **2 cups low-fat organic vanilla yogurt**
- **1 tsp vanilla extract**
- **1 tsp almond extract**
- **4 Tbsp cornstarch, dissolved in 2 Tbsp nonfat milk**
- **2 Tbsp cinnamon**
- **3 Tbsp agave nectar**
- **1 tsp orange blossom water**
- **2 Tbsp pistachios, ground**
- **4 figs**

Healthy Living Tradition

Fresh figs usually debut in the fall. In addition to eating them alone, they taste great with salads, chicken, duck, and beef and are great in baked dishes. Figs are high in fiber and contain no fat, cholesterol, or sodium.

Exchanges/Choices		Calories	250	Sodium	90mg
3 Carbohydrate		Calories from Fat	35	**Total Carbohydrate**	48g
1/2 Fat		**Total Fat**	4.0g	Dietary Fiber	4g
		Saturated Fat	1.4g	Sugars	31g
Serves 4		Trans Fat	0.0g	**Protein**	7g
Serving Size: 1/2 cup		**Cholesterol**	5mg		

Although they look like elegant chocolate truffles, these sweet treats are packed with tons of healthy nutrients. Dates have been cultivated for more than 5,000 years. This recipe can be made in advance and stored in the refrigerator for up to a week or in the freezer for up to one month.

Date, Almond, and Sesame Balls

1. Place dates, butter, 1/4 cup water, almonds, vanilla, cardamom, and cinnamon in a food processor. Pulse to form a smooth paste. Shape dough into date-size balls.

2. Spread sesame seeds on a baking sheet. Roll date balls in sesame seeds to coat. Arrange on a serving platter.

- **1 lb soft dates, pitted**
- **1/4 cup butter, at room temperature**
- **1/2 lb blanched almonds**
- **1 tsp vanilla extract**
- **1 tsp ground cardamom**
- **1/2 tsp ground cinnamon**
- **1 cup sesame seeds, toasted**

Healthy Living Tradition

Healthful no-bake desserts are wonderful beginner recipes for young children. By teaching children to make healthy recipes while they're young, they will have better eating habits as adults.

Exchanges/Choices	Calories	105	Sodium	10mg
1 Carbohydrate	Calories from Fat	55	**Total Carbohydrate**	12g
1 Fat	**Total Fat**	6.0g	Dietary Fiber	2g
	Saturated Fat	1.3g	Sugars	8g
Serves 36	Trans Fat	0.0g	**Protein**	2g
Serving Size: 1 ball	**Cholesterol**	5mg		

I invented this recipe while preparing a special dinner for my father, who loves strudel.
A few hours before the dinner, I realized I didn't have any flour left, so I decided to make it with phyllo dough instead. I added dried dates to a traditional filling to complement the Middle Eastern phyllo texture. My father ended up liking it even more than the regular version. Since then, I have taught this recipe to professional pastry chefs and home cooks in the U.S. and the Mediterranean. To make the strudel extra festive, you can use a small cookie cutter to cut out designs on the top before baking it. Be sure to thaw the phyllo dough according to package directions before beginning this recipe. Also note that this recipe contains a lot of carbohydrate, so plan your meal's carbohydrate content accordingly before eating this.

Apple, Date, and Raisin Phyllo Strudel

1. Place apples in a bowl, and cover with lemon juice.

2. To make the filling, combine 3/4 cup sugar with 1 cup water and lemon peel in a large saucepan over medium heat. Cook, stirring occasionally, until sugar has dissolved completely. Once sugar has dissolved, stop stirring. Add dates, stir to combine, and cover the saucepan. Reduce heat to low, and simmer for 20 minutes. Add apples, stir, and simmer, covered, for another 20 minutes. Remove the pan from the heat, and stir in raisins. Allow mixture to cool completely. (This step can be done a day in advance.)

2	Golden Delicious apples, peeled, cored, and cut into 1-inch pieces
1/4	cup lemon juice
3/4	cup + 1 Tbsp granulated sugar
1	(2 × 3-inch) strip lemon peel
3/4	lb dried dates, pitted and chopped into 1/2-inch pieces
1/2	cup golden raisins
7	sheets (14 × 18-inch) phyllo dough, at room temperature
4	Tbsp canola oil
3/4	cup dried plain bread crumbs

3. When mixture has cooled to room temperature, preheat the oven to 375°F. Line a baking sheet with parchment paper or a silicone liner.

4. Carefully unfold the phyllo dough, and lay one sheet down on a clean work surface. Place canola oil in a small bowl. Using a pastry brush, lightly oil the phyllo, working from the outside in. Sprinkle with 2 Tbsp bread crumbs. Continue layering phyllo dough, brushing each with oil and sprinkling with bread crumbs, until it is all gone.

5. Spoon the filling evenly down the long side of the phyllo sheet, about 2 inches from the bottom edge and 1 inch from both sides, creating a 12 × 13-inch log. Carefully fold the bottom edge and the side flaps over the filling. Slowly roll up the phyllo sheets like a jelly roll. Place on a baking sheet. Lightly brush the top of the strudel with additional canola oil. Sprinkle remaining 1 Tbsp sugar across the top. Make 16 (3/4-inch) evenly spaced diagonal slits across the top of the strudel to reveal the filling.

6. Bake for 25 minutes, and rotate pan. Bake another 10–15 minutes or until golden. Remove from the oven, and let rest for at least 10 minutes. Serve warm or at room temperature.

Healthy Living Tradition

Phyllo dough is free of trans fat, saturated fat, and cholesterol, making it an excellent alternative to butter-laden dough and crusts. Many people prefer its light, crunchy, and flaky texture, and it is perfect for soft, moist fillings. Experiment by replacing some of the traditional dough and crusts in your favorite recipes with phyllo dough.

Exchanges/Choices			
3 Carbohydrate	**Calories**	205	**Sodium** 80mg
	Calories from Fat	35	**Total Carbohydrate** 42g
	Total Fat	4.0g	Dietary Fiber 2g
Serves 16	Saturated Fat	0.3g	Sugars 28g
Serving Size: 3/4-inch slice	Trans Fat	0.0g	**Protein** 2g
	Cholesterol	0mg	
Vegan dish			

The countries of **Morocco, Tunisia, and Algeria** all serve a fabulous coil-shaped sweet called *m'hancha*, which is made out of the local phyllo-like pastry called *dioul*. This version uses easy-to-find phyllo dough and seasonal fruit for a refreshing surprise. For an extra treat, serve this with 1 Tbsp of *Yogurt Custard with Figs and Pistachios* (p. 210). Keep in mind that phyllo needs to thaw at room temperature before using.

Fruit-Filled Phyllo Snake

❋ *M'hancha* ❋

1. Combine apples, pears, agave nectar, coconut, lemon zest, almond extract, and lemon juice in a medium saucepan over medium heat. Cook for 10 minutes or until fruit is soft, stirring occasionally. Do not allow fruit to burn. Remove from heat, and set aside to cool. Stir in rose water.

2. Preheat oven to 350°F. Grease an 8-inch round baking dish with cooking spray.

3. Place canola oil in a small bowl next to a clean work surface. Lay one sheet of phyllo on a flat work surface. Brush oil over it, and top with another piece. Leaving a 1 1/2-inch border, spoon 1/4 of the apple mixture in a 1-inch line along the length of the phyllo. Pull the phyllo border over the filling to enclose and carefully roll up like a jelly roll. Place the phyllo roll in the center of the baking pan and roll into a tight coil.

3 green apples, peeled, cored, and cut into bite-size pieces
2 green pears, peeled, cored, and cut into bite-size pieces
3 Tbsp agave nectar
2 Tbsp dried unsweetened coconut
2 Tbsp lemon zest
2 tsp almond extract
   Juice of 1 lemon
1 Tbsp rose water
   Nonstick cooking spray
3 Tbsp canola oil
8 (14 × 18-inch) phyllo sheets, at room temperature
   Juice of 1 orange
1 tsp orange blossom water
1/4 cup blanched almonds, finely chopped

4. Continue brushing, filling, and rolling remaining phyllo sheets in the same manner. Wrap the subsequent rolls around the center roll to produce a tight coil formation. When all of the phyllo and filling are used, brush remaining oil over the top. Bake for 25–30 minutes or until phyllo is golden.

5. Bring orange juice and orange blossom water to a boil over medium heat. Set aside to cool. (This can be done up to a week in advance.)

6. When phyllo is done, remove from the oven, and pour orange juice mixture over the top. Invert onto a serving dish, garnish with almonds, and let cool. Serve warm or at room temperature.

Healthy Living Tradition

Agave nectar has been used as a sweetener for over 5,000 years. Agave is extracted from the heart of the blue agave plant. Available in different colors and intensities, ranging from light to amber, agave nectar can replace sugar in some recipes.

Exchanges/Choices	Calories	215	Sodium	100mg
2 Carbohydrate	Calories from Fat	80	**Total Carbohydrate**	34g
1 1/2 Fat	**Total Fat**	9.0g	Dietary Fiber	3g
	Saturated Fat	1.4g	Sugars	15g
Serves 8	Trans Fat	0.0g	**Protein**	3g
Serving Size: 1 (2-inch) piece	**Cholesterol**	0mg		

Vegan dish

This sweet breakfast dish can also be served as dessert. Served everywhere from the Middle East to India, it is popular with both children and adults. Other berries, raisins, bananas, or mixed nuts can be substituted for the strawberries.

Sweet Vermicelli with Strawberries

❋ *Sharleya bil Frawila* ❋

1. Add vermicelli, sugar, and 2 cups hot water to a medium saucepan over high heat. Bring to a boil, uncovered, over high heat. Lower heat to medium low. Simmer, uncovered, for 15–20 minutes or until vermicelli is tender. Divide vermicelli into bowls. Top each with equal portions of warm milk. Top with strawberries, and serve warm.

1 **cup vermicelli, broken into small pieces**
1/2 **cup sugar**
1/2 **cup nonfat milk, warmed**
3/4 **cup fresh strawberries, sliced**

Healthy Living Tradition

In addition to their great taste, strawberries add fiber to your diet.

Exchanges/Choices		Calories	130	Sodium	10mg
2 Carbohydrate		Calories from Fat	0	**Total Carbohydrate**	30g
		Total Fat	0.0g	Dietary Fiber	1g
Serves 6		Saturated Fat	0.1g	Sugars	19g
Serving Size: 1/2 cup		Trans Fat	0.0g	**Protein**	3g
		Cholesterol	0mg		

When I lived in Rome, one of the keys to surviving the August heat was the *granita di caffé.* Instead of a normal morning caffé latte, which is warm, I would go to the local coffee bars and order an espresso granita. Because there are only three ingredients in this recipe, the quality of the coffee determines the results. If you do not have an espresso machine, you can do as the Italians do and purchase a *moka,* a stovetop espresso maker. Most specialty grocery stores and cookware stores sell them. They are inexpensive and produce excellent results.

Espresso Granita

❊ Granita di Caffé ❊

1. Combine hot espresso with sugar in a large bowl. Whisk well until sugar dissolves. Allow the mixture to cool to room temperature. Transfer the mixture to ice cube trays to freeze. Freeze for 3–4 hours or until coffee is completely frozen.

2 cups hot espresso
1/3 cup granulated sugar
1/2 cup fat-free whipped topping
4 whole roasted espresso beans, for garnish

2. Meanwhile, chill four clear champagne flutes or other clear glasses. Place the coffee ice cubes in a food processor fitted with a metal blade or blender. Pulse on and off until the mixture is uniformly ground. Scoop the granita into the chilled cups. Top with whipped topping and a roasted espresso bean. Serve immediately.

Healthy Living Tradition

Believe it or not, a serving of espresso (1–2 oz) actually has less caffeine than a serving of regular coffee (7 oz). If you're looking to avoid caffeine altogether, choose from one of many of the decaf versions now on the market.

Exchanges/Choices		Calories	80	Sodium	20mg
1 Carbohydrate		Calories from Fat	0	Total Carbohydrate	19g
		Total Fat	0.0g	Dietary Fiber	0g
Serves 4		Saturated Fat	0.1g	Sugars	17g
Serving Size: 1/2 cup		Trans Fat	0.0g	Protein	0g
		Cholesterol	0mg		

Watermelon ice is a popular summertime treat in Italy. The Persians first brought various types of melons to ancient Rome. Melons were successfully cultivated in the town of Cantalupo, which is famous for its cantaloupes.

Watermelon and Rose Water Granita

1. In a small saucepan, combine 1/4 cup water and agave nectar. Bring to a boil, and then set aside to cool.

2. Process watermelon to a purée in a food processor, working in batches, if necessary. Combine puréed watermelon with agave nectar and rose water in a large bowl. Stir to combine.

3. Transfer mixture to a 9 × 13-inch metal baking dish, cover, and freeze for 3 hours or until frozen solid. Break up pieces of watermelon ice, and transfer to food processor. Process on and off to obtain a fine snow-like consistency. Serve in small, clear, chilled glasses or cups.

2 Tbsp agave nectar
1 1/2 lb seedless watermelon chunks, cubed
1 Tbsp rose water

Healthy Living Tradition

In addition to its thirst-quenching nature, watermelon is extremely healthy. It is low in calories, but full of vitamins C and A.

Exchanges/Choices	Calories	35	Sodium	0mg
1/2 Carbohydrate	Calories from Fat	0	**Total Carbohydrate**	9g
	Total Fat	0.0g	Dietary Fiber	0g
Serves 8	Saturated Fat	0.0g	Sugars	8g
Serving Size: 1/2 cup	Trans Fat	0.0g	**Protein**	1g
	Cholesterol	0mg		
Vegan dish				

This fruity sorbet looks as beautiful as it tastes. Sorbet is so easy to make that you'll never buy it at the store ever again.

Raspberry and Lemon Sorbet

1. Quickly wash the raspberries and place them in a blender. Purée them until they are smooth. Add the lemon juice, grape juice, and agave nectar. Purée for another minute.

2. Pass the mixture through a fine-mesh sieve, stirring and pushing the raspberry pulp down into the sieve to separate out the seeds. Place the strained mixture in a large plastic container. Put it in the freezer for 1 hour.

3. Remove the sorbet from the freezer, and spoon it back into the blender. Purée to break down the ice crystals that have formed. Freeze for another 2–3 hours or until mixture is frozen. To serve, distribute mixture in fruit glasses, and top with a lemon peel.

12	**oz fresh raspberries**
	Juice of 1/2 lemon
1/4	**cup no-sugar-added white grape juice**
1	**Tbsp blue agave nectar**
4	**thin strips lemon peel**

Healthy Living Tradition

Raspberries are a good source of vitamin C. Prior to freezing the sorbet, the purée can be used as a sauce for recipes like the Italian Sponge Cake (p. 202).

Exchanges/Choices		Calories	60	Sodium	5mg
1 Fruit		Calories from Fat	0	Total Carbohydrate	14g
		Total Fat	0.0g	Dietary Fiber	0g
Serves 4		Saturated Fat	0.0g	Sugars	9g
Serving Size: 1/2 cup		Trans Fat	0.0g	**Protein**	1g
		Cholesterol	0mg		
Vegan dish					

This light, refreshing dessert is a quick pick-me-up and a refreshing way to end a fabulous Moroccan meal. Note that an ice cream maker is needed to prepare this dish. If you do not have an ice cream maker, you can make shaved ice by freezing the juice mixture in ice cube trays and crushing the ice in a blender or food processor. I like to serve this in clear martini glasses for dramatic effect. Sorbet can be made a week ahead of time.

Moroccan Tangerine Sorbet

1. Stir juice, agave nectar, and orange blossom water together in a bowl. Cover. Chill mixture for 3–4 hours or until cold.

2. To make sorbet, freeze juice in an ice cream maker according to manufacturer's directions.

3. To serve, divide equal amounts into 10 clear cups, ramekins, or martini glasses. Garnish each with a mint sprig. Serve immediately.

18 tangerines, juiced (or enough to make 3 1/2 cups juice)
1/2 cup blue agave nectar
1 Tbsp orange blossom water
10 sprigs fresh mint

Healthy Living Tradition

Tangerines were first shipped to Europe in 1841 from the Moroccan port town of Tangiers, which how they got their English name. Tangerines were traditionally brought to Turkish steam baths. While bathers enjoyed the steam, they would peel the tangerines, releasing their intoxicating citrus aroma, and eat them to prevent dehydration. Also, a single serving of tangerine is packed with vitamin C. Why not incorporate them into your snack regimen during cold and flu season?

Exchanges/Choices	Calories	75	Sodium	10mg
1/2 Fruit	Calories from Fat	0	**Total Carbohydrate**	18g
1/2 Carbohydrate	**Total Fat**	0.0g	Dietary Fiber	0g
	Saturated Fat	0.0g	Sugars	18g
Serves 10	Trans Fat	0.0g	**Protein**	0g
Serving Size: 1/10 recipe	**Cholesterol**	0mg		

Vegan dish

This light, beautiful, and elegant dessert will suit any occasion when the color pink will be appreciated. Inspired by the Provençal dish *oeufs a la neige*, this dessert will delight your guests.

French Meringue with Rose Cream

1. Combine sugar with 1 tsp rose water in a small bowl.

2. Place 2 1/4 cups milk in a wide pan over medium heat.

3. Beat the egg whites until stiff peaks form. Set aside.

4. Using spoons, form 12 egg shapes out of the egg whites. Place on top of the hot milk as it begins to boil. (If your pan is not large enough to accommodate all 12 shapes, do this step in batches.) Carefully spoon hot milk over the egg whites to cook them. In 1–2 minutes, meringues should be poached. Lift poached meringues out of the milk with a slotted spoon. Place on a platter. Remove any bits of meringue from the milk mixture. Stir in the sugar-rose water mixture, and bring to a boil again.

5. Dissolve cornstarch in 1/4 cup milk. Slowly pour the cornstarch mixture into the pan while mixing. Allow mixture to boil until a custard-like consistency is formed (about 2 minutes). Remove pudding from flame. Stir in red food coloring, and set aside. Let cool to room temperature.

6. To serve, set out six small dessert plates or bowls. Spread 1/6 of pudding in each one. Carefully place two meringues on top of each, making sure that the pink cream shows through the meringues.

1/4 cup sugar
2 tsp rose water, divided
2 1/4 cups + 1/4 cup nonfat milk, divided
2 egg whites
2 Tbsp cornstarch
1 drop red food coloring

Healthy Living Tradition

Meringue, in addition to being a popular French dessert ingredient, is actually healthful. Egg whites contain the same amount of protein as egg yolks, yet contain fewer calories and no fat. Try making omelets and scrambled eggs from egg whites with tomatoes or roasted red peppers added for color.

Exchanges/Choices	Calories	85	Sodium	75mg
1 Carbohydrate	Calories from Fat	0	Total Carbohydrate	16g
	Total Fat	0.0g	Dietary Fiber	0g
Serves 6	Saturated Fat	0.1g	Sugars	13g
Serving Size: 2 meringues	Trans Fat	0.0g	Protein	5g
+ 1/4 cup cream	Cholesterol	0mg		

You will need eight (8-inch) bamboo skewers for serving this beautiful and edible centerpiece. As guests pull the skewers out of the orange, the orange flavor will have already penetrated the skewer for an extra burst of flavor. Try these at your next party or barbecue. They're sure to be a hit.

Grapes with Goat Cheese and Almonds

1. Remove the green grapes from the stem, and wash well.

2. In a small bowl, combine goat cheese and milk. Mix well until a creamy, icing-like consistency is formed. Transfer to a plate.

3. Place almonds on another plate.

4. Thread 6 grapes onto each skewer, leaving at least a 1-inch border from the point end. Roll each one into goat cheese mixture, using a brush or your fingers to make a thin, even coat all over the grapes. Dip the skewer into the almonds, and turn to coat. Shake off excess almonds. Set on a plate. Continue this process until all skewers are complete.

5. Cut off the bottom of an orange so it can sit flat. Stick the pointed ends of the skewers into the orange, so it looks like a bouquet. Chill until serving.

48 seedless green grapes (about 1 lb)
2 oz goat cheese
3 Tbsp nonfat milk
1/2 cup blanched almonds, coarsely ground, plus extra for garnish
1 orange, for serving

Healthy Living Tradition

Because they contain few calories, a handful of fresh, in-season grapes is an excellent snack.

Exchanges/Choices		Calories	95	Sodium	30mg
1/2 Fruit		Calories from Fat	55	**Total Carbohydrate**	8g
1 Fat		**Total Fat**	6.0g	Dietary Fiber	1g
		Saturated Fat	1.4g	Sugars	5g
Serves 8		Trans Fat	0.0g	**Protein**	4g
Serving Size: 1 kabob		**Cholesterol**	5mg		

Fromage d'affinois **is a double-cream French cheese that is produced in a manner similar** to brie. Unlike brie, however, the cow's milk goes through an ultrafiltration process, which removes all of its water content to produce a denser, more flavorful cheese. It pairs well with bread, grapes, figs, and berries. Fig jam and *fromage d'affinois* are available at most supermarkets and specialty stores.

Fig and Fromage D'Affinois Crostini

1. Toast bread until hardened but barely light gold in color. Spread 1 tsp *fromage d'affinois* on top of each piece of bread. Top with 1 tsp fig jam, and serve.

4 **thin slices of French bread (about 1 oz each)**
1 1/2 **Tbsp *fromage d'affinois***
4 **tsp Adriatic fig jam**

Healthy Living Tradition

Cheeses are popular desserts in the Mediterranean. Many people would rather forgo a sweet chocolate creation for a small piece of cheese. Although many cheeses can be fattening in large quantities, small portions can be immensely satisfying.

Exchanges/Choices				
1 1/2 Carbohydrate	**Calories**	120	**Sodium**	220mg
1/2 Fat	Calories from Fat	20	**Total Carbohydrate**	21g
	Total Fat	2.5g	Dietary Fiber	1g
	Saturated Fat	1.4g	Sugars	5g
Serves 4	Trans Fat	0.0g	**Protein**	4g
Serving Size: 1 crostini	**Cholesterol**	5mg		

Fruit soups are the perfect summertime dessert. Light, refreshing, sweet, and bursting with flavor, they end the meal with a bang. Check out your local farmer's market to make this recipe with the freshest ingredients. This soup should be made at the last minute and served immediately.

Melon, Plum, and Nectarine Soup

1. Peel and dice plums, reserving a few tablespoons. Dice nectarines. Combine with plums in a food processor with 2 cups water and agave nectar. Process until a purée is formed.

2. Pour purée through a fine-mesh sieve into a bowl, pressing on top of mixture and discarding solids.

3. Stir reserved plums, lime zest, lime juice, and watermelon into the purée. Serve immediately, garnished with mint sprigs.

- 1 lb black plums, chilled
- 1 lb nectarines, chilled
- 2 Tbsp agave nectar
  Zest of 1 lime
  Juice of 1 lime
- 1/2 cup chopped, seeded watermelon
- 4 mint sprigs

Healthy Living Tradition

When buying plums, test ripeness by gently squeezing the plum between your thumb and forefinger. If its skin is very tight, it's not ripe yet. A little bit of give means that it's ready to be eaten.

Exchanges/Choices					
2 Fruit	Calories	105	Sodium	10mg
	Calories from Fat	5	**Total Carbohydrate**	26g
	Total Fat	0.5g	Dietary Fiber	1g
Serves 4	Saturated Fat	0.0g	Sugars	22g
Serving Size: 1/4 recipe	Trans Fat	0.0g	**Protein**	2g
	Cholesterol	0mg		
Vegan dish				

At the first sight of fresh, plump nectarines at farmer's markets and roadside stands, I get the urge to make this recipe. The flavor of mint complements the color and flavor of nectarines and elevates a few humble ingredients into an extraordinary dessert. Originally from China, nectarines are grown on peach trees, yet have smooth skin and a slightly spicier flavor. Some peach trees produce both peaches and nectarines. In this recipe, the mint must be dried well, either with a salad spinner or kitchen towels, to prevent it from discoloring.

Nectarines with Mint Sugar

1. Slice nectarines into eighths, remove pits, and place slices in a large bowl. Reserve 4 whole mint sprigs, and place the rest of the mint and all of the sugar in a food processor. Pulse on and off until a paste is formed. Stir nectarines into paste, mixing well to coat. Cover. Allow flavors to blend at room temperature for a few hours or overnight in the refrigerator. To serve, place 8 nectarine slices onto a plate in the shape of a sun or flower, and place a mint sprig in the middle for garnish.

4　large, ripe (but not mushy) nectarines
1　bunch fresh mint, washed and dried well
1/4　cup natural sugar

Healthy Living Tradition

Many local orchards offer pick-your-own peach and nectarine hours. Why not get your family and friends together for this fun outing that lets you socialize, get fresh air, and exercise all at the same time?

Exchanges/Choices	Calories	120	Sodium	0mg
1 Fruit	Calories from Fat	5	**Total Carbohydrate**	29g
1 Carbohydrate	**Total Fat**	0.5g	Dietary Fiber	3g
	Saturated Fat	0.0g	Sugars	25g
Serves 4	Trans Fat	0.0g	**Protein**	2g
Serving Size: 1 nectarine (8 slices)	**Cholesterol**	0mg		

Vegan dish

Originally found only in ancient Persia (modern-day Iran), peaches were introduced to the rest of the world through the trading routes of the Silk Road. Everyday desserts in the Mediterranean region consist of fresh fruit. When fruit is at its peak, it doesn't need a lot of coaxing to taste great. The sweet, musky flavor of basil really enhances sugary peaches, while creamy yogurt cools the palate. Note that the yogurt in this recipe needs to be drained overnight. My culinary students love to serve these for brunch.

Peaches in Basil-Yogurt Cream

1. Place a colander inside a bowl. Add yogurt. Set in the refrigerator for 6 hours or overnight.

2. Preheat oven to 400°F. Grease a large baking dish with oil. Place peaches, cut side up, inside, and sprinkle 1 tsp sugar over each. Bake, uncovered, for 35 minutes.

3. While peaches are baking, stir together yogurt, basil, and honey. Divide half of yogurt mixture onto the bottom of each of four plates or a large serving platter. When peaches have finished baking, remove from the oven. Place two halves over yogurt on each plate. Fill holes with yogurt mixture, and serve warm.

1 cup low-fat vanilla yogurt, drained
1 tsp canola oil
4 ripe peaches, pitted and halved
4 tsp natural sugar
2 Tbsp finely chopped fresh basil
1 tsp honey

Healthy Living Tradition

Roasting fruit enhances their sweetness and gives them a unique texture. Serving them with yogurt and herbs makes them a work of art. Keep this in mind when planning desserts for yourself and your friends and family. Even though recipes like these are simple and healthful, their flavor is preferable to store-bought cakes and pastries.

Exchanges/Choices			
1 Fruit	Calories	110	Sodium 5mg
1/2 Carbohydrate	Calories from Fat	20	Total Carbohydrate 23g
	Total Fat	2.0g	Dietary Fiber 2g
	Saturated Fat	0.3g	Sugars 21g
Serves 4	Trans Fat	0.0g	Protein 2g
Serving Size: 1 peach	Cholesterol	0mg	

Poached fruit makes for an easy, elegant, and unexpected dessert that perfectly finishes a meal without adding unwanted fat and calories. Find dried hibiscus and rose petals in Indian, Mediterranean, or Middle Eastern markets or substitute the same quantity of *Rose Tea* (p. 242).

Poached Apples in Rose Tea

1. Combine water and sugar in a saucepan. Bring to a boil, stirring, over high heat. Remove from heat. Add hibiscus and rosebuds. Cover and steep for 5 minutes. Strain into a bowl and stir in rose water.

2. Bring a saucepan full of water to a boil over high heat. Add the whole apples, and cover with a plate on top to keep them submerged. Blanch the apples for 5 minutes or until soft. Drain, let cool, and peel.

3. Return apples to the saucepan, and cover with hibiscus and rosebud syrup. Bring to a simmer over medium-low heat, cover, and poach for 15 minutes or until apples are tender. Remove from heat. Let peaches cool to room temperature. Serve apples with syrup drizzled on top.

1 cup water
1/2 cup sugar
3 Tbsp dried hibiscus flowers
3 Tbsp dried rosebuds
1 Tbsp rose water
4 Golden Delicious apples

Healthy Living Tradition

Don't throw away the apple peel when a recipe calls for peeled apples. Apple peel is a great source of fiber.

Exchanges/Choices	Calories	155	Sodium	0mg
1 Fruit	Calories from Fat	0	**Total Carbohydrate**	40g
1 1/2 Carbohydrate	**Total Fat**	0.0g	Dietary Fiber	2g
	Saturated Fat	0.0g	Sugars	37g
Serves 4	Trans Fat	0.0g	**Protein**	0g
Serving Size: 1 apple	**Cholesterol**	0mg		

Vegan dish

This recipe calls for ripe plantains, which are different from green plantains. Ripe plantains look like larger, overly ripe bananas. Resist the temptation to discard blackened ripe plantains; the darker they get, the riper and sweeter they will be.

Sweet Fried Plantains

1. Cut ends off plantains. Make an incision down the length of each plantain. Cut each plantain into thirds. Remove peels.

2. Heat oil in a medium skillet. Add plantain slices, and mash down slightly. Cook for 2–3 minutes per side, until golden. Drizzle agave nectar over the top, and serve.

2 large plantains (about 1 lb each)
1 Tbsp canola oil
2 Tbsp blue agave nectar

Healthy Living Tradition

Plantains contain few calories and contain a lot of potassium and vitamins A and C. Plantains can also be boiled and mashed and served as an accompaniment to meat and chicken. Plantain rounds can be baked and salted and served in place of potato chips.

Exchanges/Choices	Calories		150	Sodium	10mg
2 Carbohydrate	Calories from Fat		20	**Total Carbohydrate**	35g
1/2 Fat	**Total Fat**		2.5g	Dietary Fiber	2g
	Saturated Fat		0.2g	Sugars	18g
Serves 6	Trans Fat		0.0g	**Protein**	1g
Serving Size: 1/3 plantain	**Cholesterol**		0mg		

Vegan dish

During the fall, fresh figs are plentiful throughout the Mediterranean. Extremely fertile trees produce so much of the crop that lucky tree owners often give away baskets of them as gifts. When I lived in Rome, we had fig trees in the courtyard of our apartment building. My landlord's wife would often give me large quantities. Because the line between fresh and ripe and spoiled is only a few days long for figs, housewives, bakers, and cooks have all come up with (and continue to invent) new ways to serve them. This recipe is both visually stunning and nutritious.

Fresh Figs with Raspberry Purée

1. Cut the stem off the figs, and stuff them with an almond each.

2. Make the sauce by puréeing the raspberries in a food processor or blender. Pass the purée through a fine-mesh sieve into another bowl by stirring and pushing down with a wooden spoon to extract the juice and leave the seeds behind. Stir in confectioners' sugar, if used. Divide sauce evenly between 6 white (if possible) dessert plates. Arrange figs right side up on top of sauce.

18 fresh, ripe figs
18 blanched whole almonds
1 1/2 cups fresh raspberries (frozen and thawed can be substituted)
Confectioner's sugar, if desired

Healthy Living Tradition

Figs were often linked to sexuality in Mediterranean folklore.

Exchanges/Choices		Calories	145	Sodium	0mg
2 Fruit		Calories from Fat	20	**Total Carbohydrate**	32g
1/2 Fat		**Total Fat**	2.5g	Dietary Fiber	5g
		Saturated Fat	0.3g	Sugars	26g
Serves 6		Trans Fat	0.0g	**Protein**	2g
Serving Size: 3 figs		**Cholesterol**	0mg		
+ 1 1/3 Tbsp sauce					

Vegan dish

Rose water is one of the most unique and delicious ingredients in the Mediterranean. Rose water is made from the distillation of rose oil. After Islamic alchemists perfected distillation, rose water became an indispensable ingredient in drinks and desserts everywhere, from Turkey in the east to Morocco in the west. Use whatever fresh fruit is available to make this delicious fruit salad.

Rose and Mint Infused Fruit Salad
❊ Salata bil Fakha, Ward, wa Na'na ❊

1. Combine all fruit in a large salad bowl.

2. Combine agave nectar, rose water, and mint in a small bowl.

3. Drizzle agave nectar mixture over fruit, and mix gently to combine. Cover bowl, and store in the refrigerator for at least 5 hours up to a maximum of overnight. Transfer to individual bowls before serving. Garnish with whipped cream, if desired.

- 1 cup cantaloupe, cubed
- 1/2 cup honeydew, cubed
- 1/2 cup watermelon, cubed
- 1/2 cup blueberries
- 1/2 cup sliced kiwi
- 1/4 cup agave nectar
- 1 tsp rose water
- 4 Tbsp finely chopped fresh mint
- 1 tsp fat-free whipped topping, for garnish, if desired

Healthy Living Tradition

Fresh herbs and fruit are used to create delicious weeknight desserts across the Mediterranean. Always choose items that are in season to ensure the best flavor. Mint and basil work well with most summer fruits, whereas thyme and rosemary work with roasted winter fruits.

Exchanges/Choices		Calories	65	Sodium	15mg
1/2 Fruit		Calories from Fat	0	**Total Carbohydrate**	17g
1/2 Carbohydrate		**Total Fat**	0.0g	Dietary Fiber	1g
		Saturated Fat	0.0g	Sugars	15g
Serves 6		Trans Fat	0.0g	**Protein**	1g
Serving Size: 1/2 cup		**Cholesterol**	0mg		

Vegan dish

Dramatic Drinks

"The heart seeks neither coffee nor the coffeehouse.
The heart seeks a friend—coffee is just an excuse."

—Turkish proverb

These traditional Mediterranean drink recipes are steeped in tradition and ritual. Meals and business deals are traditionally closed with coffee and tea. Throughout the region, festive occasions are celebrated with fresh fruit drinks, and healthful tisanes are dutifully prepared for ailing loved ones. The drinks of the Mediterranean can be divided into two categories: hot and cold. The hot drinks include coffee, tea, and herb and spice tisanes, which were obtained over centuries of trade. Over the years, the exchange of ingredients, recipes, and traditions fortified powerful economic, social, and culinary ties among the various countries in the region. The cold drinks include locally grown delicacies and historically provided a boost to rural economies.

It is interesting to note that the traditional drinks prepared in the region did not originally contain sugar. Sugar did not become readily available in the region until the 19th century. This is due to the fact that when the Spaniards colonized Latin America, they brought sugar cane (which was originally obtained in Persia and Egypt) with them and began cultivating it there. Imported sugar was so expensive that the French began making substitutes for it, such as beet sugar. In 18th century France, sugar was available in apothecaries instead of markets. It was used in small quantities, along with imported chocolate, coffee, and ground orchid powder, to treat illnesses. Most desserts of the time were sweetened with honey or molasses. Fresh fruit remained the most affordable and nutritious daily dessert in most countries, and it still is today.

In addition to their interesting historical roots, the traditional drinks of the Mediterranean are also some of the most healthful in the world. Most contain very little, if any, sugar, yet boast a wide variety of benefits. The oldest of the drinks, the *Yogurt Drink* (p. 233), was originally prepared by the Bedouins who inhabited North Africa and the Middle East. The Tunisians use the protein and healthy fats found in almonds in the delicious *Almond Milk Cooler* (p. 234), and the *Arabian Apricot Nectar* (p. 235) will help prevent dehydration. Teas made from *mint* (p. 240), *anise* (p. 241), and *rose* (p. 242) all aid in digestion. Learning to make these delicious drinks and understanding when to serve them to maximize their health benefits will enable you to start new, healthful, and sweet traditions in your own home.

In ancient times, yogurt was originally enjoyed by Bedouins. As they would travel across the desert, they would tie bags of milk to the backs of their camels. As the animal moved, the milk was shaken back and forth, turning it into yogurt. Drinking yogurt became popular during the hot seasons. Variations of this recipe exist everywhere in the Middle East.

Yogurt Drink

1. Place yogurt, water, mint, garlic, and salt in a large bowl. Stir together to form a liquid. Serve immediately or store in the refrigerator.

3 cups plain, fat-free yogurt
3 cups water
2 Tbsp fresh mint, finely chopped
1 clove garlic, minced
1/4 tsp kosher salt

Healthy Living Tradition

Yogurt is incredibly healthy. Look for ways to incorporate it into your diet.

Exchanges/Choices	Calories	60	Sodium	165mg
1/2 Fat-Free Milk	Calories from Fat	0	**Total Carbohydrate**	9g
	Total Fat	0.0g	Dietary Fiber	0g
Serves 6	Saturated Fat	0.1g	Sugars	8g
Serving Size: 1 cup	Trans Fat	0.0g	**Protein**	6g
	Cholesterol	10mg		

Almond milk is an extremely popular drink in Sicily and Tunisia. Sweetened versions are made when almonds are fresh. This drink can be enjoyed at any time of day.

Almond Milk Cooler

1. Bring almonds, milk, and lemon zest to a boil in a medium saucepan over medium heat. Cook for 5 minutes, and transfer to a blender. Remove the middle spout from the lid, place a towel over the hole, and purée the almond mixture until smooth. Stir in agave nectar, and add ice cubes. Process until smooth, and whip until frothy. Chill in clear glasses for an hour or until cold. Serve cold.

1 2/3 cups blanched almonds
3 cups nonfat milk
1 tsp lemon zest
3 Tbsp agave nectar
10 ice cubes

Healthy Living Tradition

If you'd like an alternative to dairy milk, try making almond milk. Combine 1 cup raw almonds with 4 cups water in a bowl, and refrigerate overnight. In the morning, stir the mixture, and strain the milk into another bowl, pressing down on the almonds to release most of the liquid. Store in an airtight container in the refrigerator.

Exchanges/Choices	Calories	200	Sodium	55mg
1/2 Fat-Free Milk	Calories from Fat	125	**Total Carbohydrate**	14g
1/2 Carbohydrate	**Total Fat**	14.0g	Dietary Fiber	3g
2 1/2 Fat	Saturated Fat	1.1g	Sugars	9g
	Trans Fat	0.0g	**Protein**	9g
Serves 9	**Cholesterol**	0mg		
Serving Size: 1/2 cup				

The Arabic term for dried apricot, *qamr din*, literally translates as "moon of faith." In the Muslim world, dried fruits and this nectar are usually served to break the fast during Ramadan. Dried apricot paste can be found in Middle Eastern and Mediterranean markets. It comes from Syria, where there were once 21 different varieties of apricots. Now there are only nine in existence.

Arabian Apricot Nectar

❋ *Assir Qamr Din* ❋

1. Break apricot paste into small (2-inch) pieces and place in a container of boiling water. Let stand at room temperature until the apricot paste has mostly dissolved. Stir the mixture with a wooden spoon to dissolve the rest. Pour into a pitcher, and refrigerate until cold.

1 (17.6-oz) package dried apricot paste
2 quarts boiling water

Healthy Living Tradition

The ancient Arabians used a mixture of mashed apricots and water to help prevent dehydration.

Exchanges/Choices		Calories	80	Sodium	0mg
1 1/2 Carbohydrate		Calories from Fat	0	Total Carbohydrate	21g
		Total Fat	0.0g	Dietary Fiber	1g
Serves 20		Saturated Fat	0.1g	Sugars	10g
Serving Size: 1/2 cup		Trans Fat	0.0g	Protein	0g
		Cholesterol	0mg		

Delicious macerated dried fruits are used in many Mediterranean drinks. Keep in mind that the raisins need to be soaked overnight before you make this drink.

Date and Raisin Drink

1. Place raisins, dates, soaking water from both, sugar, and rose water in a blender. Whip until all ingredients are combined. Place the extra raisins at the bottom of glasses. Distribute ice into each glass. Pour drink over ice. Serve immediately.

1 **cup raisins, stems removed and soaked overnight in 2 cups water, plus a few extra**

1/2 **cup dates, pitted, chopped, and soaked overnight in 2 cups water**

2 **Tbsp sugar, or to taste**

1 **Tbsp rose water**

1 **cup crushed ice**

Healthy Living Tradition

Raisins contain high levels of iron, which helps the body in treating anemia.

Exchanges/Choices	Calories	120	Sodium	10mg
2 Fruit	Calories from Fat	0	Total Carbohydrate	32g
	Total Fat	0.0g	Dietary Fiber	2g
Serves 6	Saturated Fat	0.0g	Sugars	26g
Serving Size: 3/4 cup	Trans Fat	0.0g	Protein	1g
	Cholesterol	0mg		

Orange blossom water is obtained by pressing and distilling the oil of orange blossoms. During citrus season, these fragrant flowers permeate the air. In rural areas of Morocco, many households still produce their own orange blossom water. There, this drink is a traditional refreshment.

Orange Blossom and Mint Infused Orange Juice

1. Combine orange juice, water, and orange blossom water in a pitcher. Stir to combine. Place the bunch of fresh mint inside. Cover. Refrigerate for 1–6 hours. Remove and discard mint. Divide juice equally among four glasses, and garnish with mint.

3 cups orange juice
1 cup cold water
1 Tbsp orange blossom water
1 bunch fresh mint, with 4 mint leaves reserved

Healthy Living Tradition

Citrus fruit are high in both vitamin C and dietary fiber.

Exchanges/Choices		Calories	85	Sodium	0mg
1 1/2 Fruit		Calories from Fat	0	Total Carbohydrate	19g
		Total Fat	0.0g	Dietary Fiber	0g
Serves 4		Saturated Fat	0.0g	Sugars	19g
Serving Size: 1 cup		Trans Fat	0.0g	Protein	1g
		Cholesterol	0mg		

The Arabic word for tamarind, *tamr hindi*, translated to "Indian date" in English. For this reason, many people believe that the tamarind originated in India. In reality, tamarinds come from the *tamarindus indica* tree, which is an evergreen tree native to Africa. It has been in Africa since prehistoric times and is believed to have spread to India and Asia long before recorded history. Its fruit grows in long brown shell clusters. When the shells are opened, the sour beans are eaten or pressed into juice.

Tamarind Juice

❁ Assir Tamr Hindi ❁

1. Pour tamarind syrup and water into a pitcher. Stir well to combine. Refrigerate to chill until serving. Pour over ice.

1 cup tamarind syrup
4 cups cold water
   Ice

Healthy Living Tradition

Many international cuisines have tamarind-based recipes. Tamarind syrup adds a wonderful flavor to marinades and glazes for fish and chicken dishes.

Exchanges/Choices				
2 1/2 Carbohydrate	**Calories**	140	**Sodium**	20mg
	Calories from Fat	0	**Total Carbohydrate**	36g
	Total Fat	0.0g	Dietary Fiber	0g
Serves 4	Saturated Fat	0.0g	Sugars	36g
Serving Size: 1 1/4 cups	Trans Fat	0.0g	**Protein**	0g
	Cholesterol	0mg		

Sour cherries are extremely popular in southern Italian and Turkish cuisine. The kernels from cherries, known as *mahlap* or *mahleb*, are ground and are also used in breads and sweet recipes.

Sour Cherry Lemonade

1. Place lemons, cherries, and 6 cups water in a covered pot, and bring to boil. Reduce heat. Simmer for 20 minutes. Strain liquid into a pitcher with a fine-mesh sieve, pressing fruit against the sides to release all juice. Add agave nectar, and stir to mix well. Let cool. Refrigerate until cold. Before serving, place in a blender and whip until frothy. Serve in chilled glasses garnished with mint sprigs.

2 ripe lemons, quartered
1/4 cup sour or black cherries, pitted
6 cups water
1/2 cup agave nectar
6 mint sprigs, for garnish

Healthy Living Tradition

Lemons are full of vitamin C. Egyptians drink lemon drinks year-round to stay healthy. In the winter, serve this drink hot.

Exchanges/Choices		Calories	70	Sodium	20mg
1 Carbohydrate		Calories from Fat	0	Total Carbohydrate	18g
		Total Fat	0.0g	Dietary Fiber	0g
Serves 6		Saturated Fat	0.0g	Sugars	17g
Serving Size: 3/4 cup		Trans Fat	0.0g	Protein	0g
		Cholesterol	0mg		

This is a common North African drink that is served at all hours of the day, usually before or after, but never with, a meal.

Mint Tea

❊ Shai bil Na'na ❊

1. Place loose tea in a teapot or medium saucepan. Cover with water, and bring to a medium boil over high heat. Once it boils, remove from heat, and let steep for 5 minutes. Divide mint into four equal parts. Place in teacups. Strain tea, and pour into cups over mint. Add sugar to taste. Serve warm.

4 tsp loose tea
4 cups water
1 cup fresh mint, washed thoroughly
    Sugar, to taste

Healthy Living Tradition

Discover which low-sugar drinks you enjoy most, and drink them instead of sweet drinks.

Exchanges/Choices		Calories	5	Sodium	5mg
Free food		Calories from Fat	0	Total Carbohydrate	1g
		Total Fat	0.0g	Dietary Fiber	0g
Serves 4		Saturated Fat	0.0g	Sugars	0g
Serving Size: 1/4 recipe		Trans Fat	0.0g	Protein	0g
		Cholesterol	0mg		

Anise is a very popular ingredient in after-dinner drinks in Egypt. Middle Eastern stores often sell anise in teabags, even though making it from scratch is not difficult and is less expensive.

Anise Tea

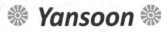 **Yansoon**

1. Bring water and anise seeds to a boil over high heat. Remove from heat. Steep, covered, for 10 minutes. Sweeten with honey, if desired. Strain into four teacups, and serve hot.

4 cups water
4 tsp dried anise seeds, slightly crushed
1 tsp honey, if desired

Healthy Living Tradition

Start a relaxing evening ritual of drinking a tisane after dinner. Decide which herbs you enjoy the most, and prepare them in the same method as above.

Exchanges/Choices		Calories	5	Sodium	10mg
Free food		Calories from Fat	0	Total Carbohydrate	1g
		Total Fat	0.0g	Dietary Fiber	0g
Serves 4		Saturated Fat	0.0g	Sugars	0g
Serving Size: 1 cup		Trans Fat	0.0g	Protein	0g
		Cholesterol	0mg		

Rose tea is a smooth, sophisticated drink made with dried rosebuds. In the Middle East and India, flower petals are fragrant culinary staples. Bags of dried rosebuds and rose water can be purchased from Middle Eastern and gourmet markets. Use your finest china for this delicate beverage.

Rose Tea

❋ *Shai bil Ward* ❋

1. Steep rosebuds and rose water, covered, in boiling water for 5 minutes. Strain, and serve hot with sugar, if desired.

4 tsp dried organic rosebuds
4 tsp rose water
4 cups boiling water
4 tsp sugar, if desired

Healthy Living Tradition

Floral teas are special and unique substitutes for caffeinated beverages.

Exchanges/Choices		Calories	0	Sodium	10mg
Free food		Calories from Fat	0	Total Carbohydrate	0g
		Total Fat	0.0g	Dietary Fiber	0g
Serves 4		Saturated Fat	0.0g	Sugars	0g
Serving Size: 1 cup		Trans Fat	0.0g	**Protein**	0g
		Cholesterol	0mg		

Ginger came to the Mediterranean from India during the spice trades. In India, Ayurvedic doctors use ginger to activate the body's fire element, which in turn burns up toxins. In foods, its zingy, warm flavor is added to soups, cookies, stews, and beverages.

Ginger Tea

1. Place ginger in boiling water. Let steep, covered, for 10 minutes. Remove lid, strain tea into teacups, and sweeten with honey, if desired.

4 tsp ground ginger or gingerroot
4 cups boiling water
1 tsp honey, optional

Healthy Living Tradition

Try incorporating 1 tsp dried ginger or freshly grated gingerroot into your favorite broth-based soup and stew recipes. It will add great flavor and health benefits.

Exchanges/Choices				
Free food	**Calories**	5	**Sodium**	10mg
	Calories from Fat	0	**Total Carbohydrate**	1g
	Total Fat	0.0g	Dietary Fiber	0g
Serves 4	Saturated Fat	0.0g	Sugars	0g
Serving Size: 1 cup	Trans Fat	0.0g	**Protein**	0g
	Cholesterol	0mg		

In Turkey, tea is enjoyed morning, noon, and night, which may explain why Turkey is a top consumer of tea in the world. Turks prefer special blends of Ceylon teas, which are renowned for their golden hue and strong flavor. For breakfast, glasses of half black tea and half warm milk are served. Black tea is usually served in short, clear tulip-shaped glasses in restaurants and coffee shops or in fine porcelain in homes. Served in beautiful samovars, drinking tea in Turkey is a national past time. There are even tea gardens, where people bring their own pastries and sit and drink tea with their families.

Black Tea with Mint

❂ *Shai bil Na'na* ❂

1. Place tea in boiling water, and add sugar, if desired. Cover, add mint, and let steep for 10 minutes for strong tea or 5 minutes for regular-strength tea. Strain tea, and pour into glasses.

4 tsp high-quality loose-leaf black tea

4 cups boiling water
  Sugar, if desired

4 sprigs fresh mint

Healthy Living Tradition

Tea contains many antioxidants, which can help keep you healthy.

Exchanges/Choices		Calories	5	Sodium	5mg
Free food		Calories from Fat	0	Total Carbohydrate	1g
		Total Fat	0.0g	Dietary Fiber	0g
Serves 4		Saturated Fat	0.0g	Sugars	0g
Serving Size: 1/4 recipe		Trans Fat	0.0g	Protein	0g
		Cholesterol	0mg		

Although Turkey is internationally renowned for its coffee, government programs implemented during the 1950s to increase tea production and boost the economy in the Black Sea region have caused production and consumption to soar. Turkish tea is served in clear, tulip-shaped crystal glasses. Serve with *Mini Turkish Sesame Bread Rings* (p. 272).

Turkish Tea

1. Place tea in boiling water. Cover, and let steep for 10 minutes. Stir in sugar, if desired. Strain tea, and pour into glasses.

4 tsp high-quality loose-leaf black tea
4 cups boiling water
  Sugar, if desired

Healthy Living Tradition

Black tea is the second most commonly drunk beverage in the world. Water is number one. In addition to tasting great, black tea is believed to have immunity-boosting properties. It also contains less caffeine than coffee.

Exchanges/Choices					
Free food	Calories	5	Sodium	5mg
	Calories from Fat	0	Total Carbohydrate	1g
	Total Fat	0.0g	Dietary Fiber	0g
Serves 4	Saturated Fat	0.0g	Sugars	0g
Serving Size: 1 cup	Trans Fat	0.0g	**Protein**	0g
	Cholesterol	0mg		

One sip of this brings me back to the open-air coffeehouses of Egypt. This is a popular after-dinner and bedtime drink in Egypt, where cinnamon is extremely popular. Egyptian cinnamon is pure cinnamon, and it tastes mellower than American cinnamon. Many Egyptian and Middle Eastern markets sell Egyptian cinnamon in teabags to make the drink instantly.

Egyptian Cinnamon Tea

✹ *Irfa* ✹

1. Combine cinnamon sticks with 4 cups water in a medium saucepan. Bring to a boil, reduce heat to low, and let simmer for 10 minutes or until the cinnamon sticks open and release their aroma. Remove cinnamon sticks, add sugar, and stir well. Pour liquid into teacups, and top each one with 1 tsp mixed nuts.

4 **cinnamon sticks**
4 **cups water**
4 **tsp sugar, or to taste**
4 **tsp mixed, dry-roasted, unsalted nuts, chopped**

Healthy Living Tradition

This tea also tastes great with hot or steamed milk; I call them cinnamon lattés. They're a great alternative for those cutting back on caffeinated drinks, like coffee and tea.

Exchanges/Choices	Calories	35	Sodium	10mg
1/2 Carbohydrate	Calories from Fat	15	**Total Carbohydrate**	5g
	Total Fat	1.5g	Dietary Fiber	0g
Serves 4	Saturated Fat	0.2g	Sugars	4g
Serving Size: 1 cup	Trans Fat	0.0g	**Protein**	0g
	Cholesterol	0mg		

Most Italians start and end their day with a cup of espresso. Coffee drinking has become an important ritual in Italian culture. Italian friends will offer each other an espresso to celebrate all aspects of life—promotions, transfers, marriages, engagements, business deals, and more. For the home, they use stovetop espresso pots called *mokas*. This recipe describes how to make delicious espresso at home using a *moka*. Gourmet and kitchenware shops often stock them in the U.S. A cup of espresso requires 40 coffee beans, and experts say that the ideal heat at which to brew espresso is the flame of a match! With that in mind, be sure to brew your espresso slowly, so it produces a light brown foam on the top known as *crema*.

Classic Italian Espresso

1. Holding the handle of the *moka* with your thumb, turn the top portion counter-clockwise to open. Lift out the basket. Fill the bottom of the *moka* about 3/4 full of cold, filtered water or to just underneath the knob on the side. Place casket back in the bottom of the *moka*, and fill with ground coffee. Carefully twist the top back on, making sure that it is positioned properly. Place *moka* over the lowest flame possible.

2. Let brew over heat for 5–7 minutes or until steam begins to come out of the spout. Remove from heat, and set aside. Pour espresso into demitasse cups, and serve hot.

6 demitasse cups
3 Tbsp ground Arabica coffee beans
Sugar, if desired

Healthy Living Tradition

A demitasse of espresso contains about half of the caffeine of a regular-size cup of brewed coffee. However, per ounce, espresso packs at least twice the amount of caffeine as brewed, drip coffee. If you enjoy coffee, try drinking espresso. The more intense coffee flavor in a small serving makes drinking it a pleasure.

Exchanges/Choices		Calories	0	Sodium	10mg
Free food		Calories from Fat	0	Total Carbohydrate	0g
		Total Fat	0.0g	Dietary Fiber	0g
Serves 6		Saturated Fat	0.1g	Sugars	0g
Serving Size: 1 demitasse		Trans Fat	0.0g	Protein	0g
(about 1.5 oz)		Cholesterol	0mg		

The Italian city of Turin is famous for its chocolate and coffee. A famous café, Caffé al Bicerin (founded in Turin in 1763), began serving exotic ingredients, like chocolate, coffee, and orange juice. Some believe that this drink was invented at this little café. When I need inspiration in the cold, winter months, I turn to a *bicerin*. I have replaced the traditional whipped cream with frothed steamed milk, and I serve it in small, clear, stemmed glasses (champagne flutes work well). If you don't have a cappuccino maker in your home you can use a portable milk frother to create foam on top. Serve this drink to guests with *Tuscan Cantucci Cookies* (p. 199) or *Anise Biscuits* (p. 195).

Bicerin

1. Divide espresso equally among four glasses.

2. Bring 1 cup nonfat milk, cocoa powder, salt, vanilla, and sugar to a boil in a saucepan over medium heat. Stir well, and whisk to combine. Pour this chocolate mixture over espresso in glasses.

3. Heat remaining 1/2 cup milk over medium heat, and with a portable milk frother, froth milk into a foamy consistency. Divide milk among the four glasses, and garnish with a dash of cinnamon.

4	**demitasses of fresh** Classic Italian Espresso (p. 247), **about 6 oz total**
1 1/2	**cups nonfat milk, divided**
2	**Tbsp cocoa powder**
	Dash salt
1/4	**tsp vanilla**
2	**Tbsp sugar**
	Dash cinnamon

Healthy Living Tradition

Did you know that dark cocoa, originally from Mexico, was first sold in apothecary shops as a medicine in Europe?

Exchanges/Choices	Calories	70	Sodium	65mg
1/2 Fat-Free Milk	Calories from Fat	5	Total Carbohydrate	13g
1/2 Carbohydrate	**Total Fat**	0.5g	Dietary Fiber	1g
	Saturated Fat	0.3g	Sugars	11g
Serves 4	Trans Fat	0.0g	**Protein**	4g
Serving Size: 1/4 recipe	**Cholesterol**	0mg		

Sufi clerics were responsible for transporting coffee from its native Ethiopia to Yemen, Saudi Arabia, and Egypt. Its taste and stimulant properties were appreciated by Imams (Muslim prayer leaders), who would drink coffee to stay awake for long hours of prayer and study. The Turks obtained coffee from Egypt and sold it to Europeans. By the 16th century, drinking coffee was an important ritual throughout the Mediterranean. A *cezve* (a small, long-handled pot with a spout) is used to prepare the coffee on the stove. If you do not have this kind of coffee pot, it can be brewed in a saucepan with a spout. Small espresso (demitasse) cups are used to serve the coffee. Ask your guests how much sugar they would like before making the coffee because the sugar is brewed in the coffee, not stirred in later.

Turkish Coffee with Cardamom

✸ Ahwa bil Habbahan ✸

1. Bring water, cardamom, and coffee to a boil in an Arabic coffee pot or saucepan. As coffee begins to boil, remove from the heat so that it does not boil over. Remove foam from the top of the coffee with a teaspoon. Place foam in the bottom of each demitasse. Let coffee stand for 1 minute off of the flame. Place pot back on the flame. When coffee begins to boil again, remove it from the heat. Let stand 1 minute off of the flame. Return coffee to flame, add desired amount of sugar, and stir. Bring to a boil a third time, but *do not* stir. Discard cardamom, and pour coffee into cups.

4 **demitasses of cold water (about 6 oz)**
1 **green cardamom pod, crushed**
4 **tsp Turkish coffee grounds**
   Sugar, to taste, if desired

Healthy Living Tradition

Life's largest problems are often solved over cups of coffee shared between friends and family in the Middle East. Developing a strategy for "face time" with our closest friends is important for our mental health and well-being.

Exchanges/Choices					
Free food	Calories	5	Sodium	0mg
	Calories from Fat	0	**Total Carbohydrate**	0g
	Total Fat	0.0g	Dietary Fiber	0g
Serves 4	Saturated Fat	0.0g	Sugars	0g
Serving Size: 1 demitasse	Trans Fat	0.0g	**Protein**	0g
(about 1.5 oz)	**Cholesterol**	0mg		

Bountiful Breads and Savory Baked Goods

One of my favorite food memories is walking through the historic center of my ancestral homeland of Crotone, Italy, on a Sunday morning with the smell of baking bread in the air. I've yet to experience a scent that is as warm, inviting, and intoxicating as fresh bread. I recently learned that I'm not alone in my love of the aroma. An old real estate trick is to bake something (even if it's from a box) in the oven of a home that is for sale during the open house. Researchers have found that buyers find homes more inviting and are likely to buy them when the aroma of freshly baking bread is in the air.

Although carbohydrates were once considered taboo for people with diabetes, nutritionists now recommend that people with diabetes consume carbohydrates in small quantities as part of a healthy diet. Many store-bought breads, however, are full of additives, sugars, and preservatives. Over the years, I have developed a passion for baking in order to duplicate some of the delicious baked goods and breads that I've enjoyed abroad in my own home. With a little advance planning, you'll be able to enjoy making baked goods from scratch as well.

One of the easiest ways to incorporate homemade breads and baked goods into a busy lifestyle is to view making them as a fun activity instead of a chore. Get excited about the positive impact that making homemade baked goods will have on your health and quality of life. Many people are amazed at how much more fulfilling a single portion of homemade bread is compared with several portions of store-bought varieties. I like to decide which breads and baked goods I'm going to make each month. Then I set aside a half day—whether morning, noon, or night—to make many different kinds of treats. I freeze what I'll be using later. In addition to producing top-notch artisan-style breads at a fraction of what they would cost at the supermarket, I enjoy myself in the process.

Baking time can be a wonderful escape from the mundane. Like sculpting clay, kneading and shaping bread dough is extremely therapeutic. Performing the same movements repeatedly leads to a Zen-like state of relaxation and calm. Baking from scratch can also be a powerful link to our past—just think back to when everyone *had* to bake from scratch. Interestingly, bread-making techniques are the same as they were in antiquity. Hundreds of varieties of breads (which look very similar to our modern breads) were being produced as early as the third millennia in Egypt. With all of the marvelous kitchen gadgets and appliances on the market today, as well as quality ingredients from around the globe, there's never been a better time to bake.

My grandmother developed a method for making this rustic, round loaf in a food processor so it doesn't need kneading. This bread is great for sandwiches, bruschetta, toast, and croutons.

Whole-Wheat French Boule Bread

1. Combine yeast and water in a large mixing bowl. Let sit for 5 minutes or until frothy. Add salt and 1 Tbsp olive oil. Mix well.

2. Place flour, 1 cup at a time, in a food processor. Slowly pulse the mixture while adding the liquid through the spout. Process until the mixture forms a ball.

3. Turn dough out onto a lightly floured surface. Form into a round loaf. Take a 9-inch cake pan, and grease it with 1 Tbsp olive oil. Sprinkle pan with cornmeal. Put rounded loaf into pan.

4. Cover with a kitchen towel, and place in an oven set on the "proof" setting (100°F). Let dough rise for 1 hour or until doubled. Remove from oven, and score the top with a knife.

5. Preheat oven to 375°F. Sprinkle *Herbes de Provence* on top of bread, and press down lightly. Bake for 25–30 minutes or until golden.

1 Tbsp active dry yeast
1 cup lukewarm water
1 tsp kosher or sea salt
2 Tbsp extra-virgin olive oil, divided
3 cups whole-wheat flour
1 Tbsp cornmeal
1 tsp Herbes de Provence (p. 277)

Healthy Living Tradition

For added texture and taste, mist the inside of the preheated oven with water just before baking this bread.

Exchanges/Choices		Calories	190	Sodium	245mg
2 Starch		Calories from Fat	40	**Total Carbohydrate**	34g
1 Fat		**Total Fat**	4.5g	Dietary Fiber	6g
		Saturated Fat	0.6g	Sugars	0g
Serves 8		Trans Fat	0.0g	**Protein**	7g
Serving Size: 1-inch slice		**Cholesterol**	0mg		

Once upon a time, country breads were made out of natural leaveners, similar to American sourdough bread. Without the addition of yeast, simple flour and water would be used as "starters." Allowed to ripen over a series of days, the starter would develop deep malty flavors and interesting texture. Before the bread was shaped, a small piece of dough would be reserved to "start" the next loaf. Although this bread is very simple to make, the entire process takes eight days, but only a few minutes each day is spent developing the dough. Making this bread with children is the perfect way to teach them about chemistry, baking, nutrition, and history all at once.

French Country Bread

Day 1

1. Place flour in a small bowl. Add water, and combine. Knead to form a dough, and cover with plastic wrap. Set aside for 2 days.

1/2 cup white whole-wheat flour
1/4 cup lukewarm water

Days 2–3

Dough is set aside

Day 4

1. Place mixture in a large bowl. Mix in lukewarm water and flour. Knead for 5 minutes to form a dough, cover with plastic wrap, and set aside.

1/2 cup lukewarm water
3/4 cup white whole-wheat flour

Day 5

1. Mix in lukewarm water. Alternate adding the flours, mixing in a little at a time to form a dough. Cover, and let rise.

1/2 cup lukewarm water
1 cup unbleached white bread flour
1/4 cup white whole-wheat flour

Days 6–8

1. Gradually mix in the final 1 cup lukewarm water, bread flour, and salt. Turn out onto a lightly floured work surface. Knead for 5–10 minutes or until smooth.

2. Grease a large bowl with the olive oil, place dough inside, and turn to coat. Cover. Let rise overnight or until doubled.

3. Knock the dough down, and shake it into a ball. Place it on a lightly floured baking sheet. Cover with a kitchen towel. Let rise overnight.

4. Preheat the oven to 500°F. Make slash marks on the top of the dough, and sprinkle with a little flour. Bake for 30 minutes, or until golden.

1 cup lukewarm water
3 cups unbleached white bread flour, plus extra for work surface
2 tsp kosher salt
2 Tbsp extra-virgin olive oil

Healthy Living Tradition

White whole-wheat flour can be found in most grocery stores. It contains 100% of the wheat germ and bran of whole-wheat flour but is much lighter in color and taste.

Exchanges/Choices		Calories	255	Sodium	325mg
3 Starch		Calories from Fat	30	**Total Carbohydrate**	47g
1/2 Fat		**Total Fat**	3.5g	Dietary Fiber	3g
		Saturated Fat	0.4g	Sugars	1g
Serves 12		Trans Fat	0.0g	**Protein**	8g
Serving Size: 1 slice		**Cholesterol**	0mg		

This simple recipe is rewarding to prepare and eat. You can substitute the unbleached bread flour for white whole-wheat flour if you prefer. If you do not have time to wait for the dough to rise, you can cover it tightly and allow it to rise for 24 hours in the refrigerator. On the next day, you can punch it down, shape it, and bake it.

Rustic Dinner Rolls

1. Line two baking sheets with silicone liners or parchment paper. Combine the flour, salt, and sugar in a large bowl, and make a well in the center.

2. Combine the yeast with the milk, and stir until dissolved. Pour the yeast mixture into the flour mixture. Let sit for 20 minutes or until bubbly. Add the water, and stir to form a soft dough. Transfer to a lightly floured work surface. Knead for 5–10 minutes or until dough is smooth and elastic.

3. Oil a bowl with the olive oil, and place dough in it. Turn to coat. Cover the bowl with oiled plastic wrap. Let rise for 1 1/2–2 hours or until doubled in size. (This step can also be done overnight in the refrigerator. You can leave it for about 20 hours.)

4. After dough has risen, place it back on a work surface, and punch it down to deflate it. Let the dough rest for 15 minutes. Roll the dough into a log, and break off 12 equal pieces. Shape each piece into balls by cupping your hand around the ball on a work surface and then rolling it into an oval. Space the rolls 2 inches apart on baking sheets, and sprinkle lightly with flour. Cover with lightly oiled plastic wrap. Let rise for another 30 minutes.

3 1/2 **cups unbleached bread flour, plus extra for work surface**
1 **tsp kosher salt**
1 **tsp sugar**
4 1/2 **tsp active dry yeast**
1/2 **cup lukewarm nonfat milk**
1 **cup lukewarm water**
1 **Tbsp extra-virgin olive oil**

5. Remove plastic wrap, and oil the side of your pinky finger with olive oil. Make slits down the middle of each roll by pressing the side of your hand into them. Let rest for 15 minutes.

6. Preheat the oven to 450°F. Place a baking pan filled with a cup of water in the bottom of the oven. Place rolls in the center rack, and bake for 15–20 minutes or until lightly golden. Serve warm, or place in large plastic storage bags and freeze until needed.

Healthy Living Tradition

Not only is homemade bread more wholesome and free of unwanted chemicals, fillers, and sugars, it's also deeply satisfying to make and provides a workout for the upper arms. The next time you have too many worries on your mind, try making homemade bread. You'll be relaxed and comforted in no time.

Exchanges/Choices	Calories	175	Sodium	170mg
2 Starch	Calories from Fat	20	**Total Carbohydrate**	33g
	Total Fat	2.0g	Dietary Fiber	1g
Serves 12	Saturated Fat	0.2g	Sugars	2g
Serving Size: 1 roll	Trans Fat	0.0g	**Protein**	6g
	Cholesterol	0mg		

If you walk through any market in the Middle East, you'll see people carrying large stacks of bread on trays on top of their heads. Most people living in the region usually buy their bread directly from the baker. Because fresh bread is so easily accessible, it is not usually made at home. If you're used to buying pre-made pita bread, I urge you to try this recipe when you have the time. You can double it and freeze the leftovers. When needed, thaw the bread and heat it under the broiler.

Whole-Wheat Pita Bread

❋ *Khubz* ❋

1. Add flours, yeast, olive oil, water, and salt to a bowl fitted to an electric mixer. Combine with the mixer or by hand. Once the ingredients are incorporated, knead the dough for 20 minutes by hand or for 3 minutes with a standing mixer using the dough hook on medium speed.

2. Oil a bowl with about 1 tsp olive oil. Add dough and let rest for 45 minutes, uncovered.

3. Sprinkle a clean work surface and two large baking sheets with the additional whole-wheat flour. Roll the dough into an even log with your hands. Cut it into 10 equal pieces. Form 10 circles with your hands or roll out with a rolling pin to shape 10 round pita breads. Place four to six pitas on each baking sheet. Let rest for 30 minutes.

4. Preheat the broiler. Place bread in oven, and bake for 2–3 minutes per side, until puffed and golden. Serve warm.

1 1/4 cups unbleached bread flour
3/4 cup whole-wheat flour, plus extra for work surface
1 tsp active dry yeast
1/2 tsp olive oil, plus 1 tsp extra for oiling a bowl
3/4 cup lukewarm water
1/2 tsp sea salt or kosher salt

Healthy Living Tradition

Place extra bread in a plastic bag while still warm, and seal it to prevent the bread from drying out.

Exchanges/Choices	Calories	110	Sodium	120mg
1 1/2 Starch	Calories from Fat	10	**Total Carbohydrate**	21g
	Total Fat	1.0g	Dietary Fiber	2g
Serves 10	Saturated Fat	0.1g	Sugars	0g
Serving Size: 1 pita	Trans Fat	0.0g	**Protein**	4g
	Cholesterol	0mg		

This rustic, simple bread is unique to the Liguria region of northwestern Italy. Known for Genoa's famed past as a port on the spice routes, the region boasts many "unexpected" ingredients in its local cuisine, chickpea flour being one of them. This bread is baked in a *testo*—a tin-plated copper pan— underneath a fire. I find that baking this bread under the broiler is the best way to duplicate a direct flame.

Italian Chickpea Flour Bread

✳ Farinata ✳

1. Place the flour, salt, olive oil, and water in a large bowl. Stir to combine. Let the mixture rest for at least 2 hours.

2. Grease a cookie sheet with a little olive oil. After the mixture has rested, stir the mixture again, and pour it into the baking sheet. Preheat the broiler, and bake for 15–20 minutes with the door left slightly ajar. Serve hot, with a sprinkle of freshly ground black pepper.

1 **cup chickpea flour**
3/4 **tsp kosher salt**
2 **Tbsp extra-virgin olive oil**
1 1/2 **cups water**
Freshly ground black pepper, to taste

Healthy Living Tradition

Chickpea flour is a great gluten-free substitute for regular flour. It also thickens sauces quickly. It is available at most Indian and import stores.

Exchanges/Choices	Calories		150	Sodium	380mg
1 Starch	Calories from Fat		70	Total Carbohydrate	13g
1 1/2 Fat	Total Fat		8.0g	Dietary Fiber	2g
	Saturated Fat		1.1g	Sugars	2g
Serves 4	Trans Fat		0.0g	Protein	5g
Serving Size: 1/4 recipe	Cholesterol		0mg		

Focaccia **is a northern Italian word that refers to a creation that comes from fire.** In some areas of Italy, *focaccia* is known as *pizza bianca*. During the grape harvest, it is studded with grapes and referred to as *schiacciata*. The traditional Genovese version of focaccia requires making a sponge first, but this is a more straightforward method. Use this focaccia to make sandwiches, or cut it into thin strips and serve with dinner. Wrap leftovers in plastic wrap and foil and freeze.

Rosemary Focaccia

1. Dissolve yeast in 1/4 cup water in a small bowl. Let stand 10 minutes or until bubbly.

2. Put flour and salt into a large bowl, and make a well in the center. Add yeast mixture and 1 cup lukewarm water. Mix well to incorporate, and form a ball. Stir in 2 Tbsp olive oil. If dough is too sticky, add a little more flour, a tablespoon at a time. If dough is too dry, add more water, a tablespoon at a time.

3. Lightly dust a work surface with flour. Knead dough for 10 minutes or until smooth and elastic.

1	package active dry yeast or 2 1/2 tsp loose yeast
1 1/4	cups lukewarm water, divided
3 1/2	cups unbleached, all-purpose flour, plus extra for work surface
1	tsp kosher or sea salt
5	Tbsp extra-virgin olive oil, divided
2	Tbsp polenta or other cornmeal
2	Tbsp fresh rosemary, finely chopped

4. Oil a large bowl with 1 Tbsp olive oil. Place dough inside, and turn to coat. Cover with a few kitchen towels, and let rise for 1 1/2 hours, until doubled in size. After dough has risen, knock it back. Divide into two balls.

5. Place on a lightly floured work surface and, with a floured rolling pin, roll out into two (1-inch-thick) oblongs. Using your fingers, make dimples all over the dough. Brush dough with remaining 2 Tbsp olive oil. Sprinkle two baking sheets with 1 Tbsp polenta each. Place one focaccia on each sheet.

6. Preheat oven to 425°F. Cover baking sheets loosely with foil, and let rise for 30 minutes. Sprinkle focaccia with rosemary, and bake 20–25 minutes or until golden. Let cool slightly before serving.

Healthy Living Tradition

Herbalists in the Mediterranean sell numerous products made from rosemary. Try growing a rosemary plant and cooking with rosemary on a regular basis for great-tasting flavors.

Exchanges/Choices	Calories	205	Sodium	160mg
2 Starch	Calories from Fat	55	**Total Carbohydrate**	32g
1 Fat	**Total Fat**	6.0g	Dietary Fiber	1g
	Saturated Fat	0.8g	Sugars	1g
Serves 12	Trans Fat	0.0g	**Protein**	4g
Serving Size: 1/12 loaf	**Cholesterol**	0mg		

This simple, homey bread is an Algerian Berber classic. The tradition of making it in a shallow baking tin, called a *gas'aa* or *tagine*, gives it a crunchy exterior and moist crumb—perfect for sopping up sauces and stews. Numerous versions of this bread abound, and it can be made on the stovetop, over an open flame, or in the oven. To get the proper texture without purchasing special equipment, I bake the bread in a 9-inch square cast-iron pan. Semolina is made from the part of the wheat berry that is between the outer bran layer and the inner layer. Finely ground cornmeal can be substituted for the semolina, if desired.

Algerian Skillet Bread

❋ *Khubz Matloua* ❋

1. Dissolve the yeast in 1/4 cup lukewarm water. Set aside for 5 minutes. Combine the semolina and salt. Stir into the yeast mixture. Add remaining 1 1/4 cups water. Stir well to combine.

2. Lightly flour a work surface, and turn dough out onto it. Knead for 5–10 minutes or until dough is supple and forms a ball. Return dough to bowl, cover with oiled plastic wrap, and let rise 1 1/2 hour or until doubled in size.

- **2 Tbsp active dry yeast**
- **1 1/2 cups lukewarm water, divided**
- **4 cups fine semolina**
- **1 tsp salt**
  Unbleached, all-purpose flour, for work surface
  Olive oil, for oiling plastic wrap

3. Preheat oven to 425°F. Lightly flour a 9-inch cast-iron skillet or other 9-inch baking pan. Punch down the dough, and place it inside the skillet or pan. Lightly wet your fingertips, and press down on the dough to evenly fill the skillet. Bake for 20–25 minutes or until lightly golden and bread pulls away from the sides of the pan. Let cool for at least 15 minutes before cutting.

Healthy Living Tradition

Fresh-baked breads like this one contain only a handful of healthful ingredients, instead of paragraphs full of unidentifiable ones found on commercially prepared bread. Baking bread is an extremely pleasurable activity that uses all of the senses. For your next gathering with children, plan on teaching them how to make easy bread recipes like this. You'll be passing on not only an important tradition, but a healthy and inexpensive hobby as well.

Exchanges/Choices		Calories	165	Sodium	145mg
2 Starch		Calories from Fat	5	Total Carbohydrate	33g
		Total Fat	0.5g	Dietary Fiber	2g
Serves 16		Saturated Fat	0.1g	Sugars	0g
Serving Size: 1 slice		Trans Fat	0.0g	**Protein**	6g
		Cholesterol	0mg		

Fougasse **is a popular bread in the south of France.** Believed to have been used to test oven temperatures, it also became popular in Corsica, when the French gained control of it. Before baking, the *fougasse* is slashed with four deep incisions and stretched apart, making it look like a ladder. Its soft crumb, rich flavor, and attractive aesthetics will impress your guests.

Corsican Olive Bread

✿ *Fougasse* ✿

1. Dissolve yeast in 1/4 cup lukewarm water. Set aside for 5 minutes.

2. Sift together flour and salt in a large bowl, and make a well in the center. Pour the yeast into the flour mixture. Stir to combine. Stir in 1 Tbsp olive oil and remaining water. Mix well to create a soft dough. If dough is too sticky, add more flour, a tablespoon at a time. If dough is too dry, add more water, a tablespoon at a time. Turn out onto a lightly floured work surface, and knead for 8–10 minutes or until soft.

3. Oil a bowl with 1 Tbsp olive oil. Place dough inside, and turn to coat. Cover with lightly oiled plastic wrap and a kitchen towel. Let rest for 1 hour or until doubled in bulk.

4. After it has risen, turn dough out onto a lightly floured surface, and knock it back. Divide dough into two pieces. With a floured rolling pin, roll dough out into two (11 × 6-inch) ovals.

5. Combine olives, sage, and capers. Scatter half over each oval. Roll dough up over filling, and create a ball. Slowly roll each ball back out into the same-size oblongs. Transfer each oblong to a baking sheet. Make four deep, diagonal, equally spaced slits (creating holes), leaving the borders intact. Gently pull the dough at opposite ends to open the slits and create wider holes. Brush each oblong with 1 Tbsp olive oil. Cover each loosely with plastic wrap. Let rest for 20 minutes.

6. Preheat oven to 425°F. Bake for 15–20 minutes or until golden. Let cool slightly before eating.

2 1/4	tsp active dry yeast
1 1/2	cups lukewarm water, divided
4	cups unbleached bread flour, plus extra for work surface
1	tsp sea salt, preferably grey
4	Tbsp extra-virgin olive oil, divided
1/3	cup niçoise olives, pitted and chopped
2	Tbsp fresh sage, finely chopped
2	Tbsp capers, drained and rinsed

Healthy Living Tradition

Artisanal breads like this one make beautiful edible gifts and centerpieces. The next time you're invited to someone's home, make this delicious bread to take along as a gift. Your gift of time and energy, not to mention the flavor, will be greatly appreciated.

Exchanges/Choices		Calories	135	Sodium	160mg
1 1/2 Starch		Calories from Fat	30	**Total Carbohydrate**	22g
1/2 Fat		**Total Fat**	3.5g	Dietary Fiber	1g
		Saturated Fat	0.4g	Sugars	1g
Serves 20 (2 loaves)		Trans Fat	0.0g	**Protein**	4g
Serving Size: 1 slice		**Cholesterol**	0mg		

This easy bread has a soft, moist crumb. Although it is a Moroccan recipe, it's a great bread to have with any meal. It is best eaten the day it is made. This bread can be frozen, though. Wrap it in plastic wrap and then foil. Thaw at room temperature. Reheat in a preheated 350°F oven before serving. Humidity can affect how much flour this recipe requires, which is why there is a variable amount of flour in the ingredients list.

Moroccan Country Bread

❋ *Khubz Maghrebi* ❋

1. Pour 2 1/2 cups warm water into the large bowl of a standing electric mixer. Sprinkle yeast over water, and stir until dissolved. Add salt. Gradually stir in 6–8 cups of flour, one cup at a time, until dough pulls away from the side of the bowl.

2. Roll the dough into a 12-inch log. Shape dough into three 4-inch, dome-shaped loaves. Place loaves on a large baking sheet sprinkled with semolina. Cover with a kitchen towel, and place in a draft-free area to rise. Let rise for 1 hour or until doubled in size.

3. Preheat oven to 350°F. Uncover loaves. Brush with 1 tsp olive oil each. Bake for 20–30 minutes or until lightly golden. Let cool slightly, and serve warm.

2 1/2	cups warm water
1	Tbsp active dry yeast
1	tsp kosher salt
6–8	cups all-purpose, unbleached flour
2	Tbsp semolina
3	tsp extra-virgin olive oil

Healthy Living Tradition

People in the Mediterranean view bread as more than just a nutritional staple. Homemade bread is seen as a gift for the palate and the senses. Because this recipe makes three loaves, you can give one away and keep two for yourself.

Exchanges/Choices		Calories	120	Sodium	65mg
1 1/2 Starch		Calories from Fat	10	**Total Carbohydrate**	24g
		Total Fat	1.0g	Dietary Fiber	1g
Serves 30 (3 loaves, about		Saturated Fat	0.1g	Sugars	1g
10 slices per loaf)		Trans Fat	0.0g	**Protein**	3g
Serving Size: 1 slice		**Cholesterol**	0mg		

Fatayer **are tender bread triangles stuffed with spinach, cheese, or meat.** They originated in Lebanon and can be found in bakeries, street stalls, and home kitchens. They are a delightful snack to enjoy anytime, but are also served as special appetizers for holiday occasions. I always bake a large batch of these delicious little breads so that I can freeze them. Whenever I need to, I can defrost them and reheat them in the oven.

Spinach-Stuffed Bread Triangles
❊ *Fatayer bil Sabanikh* ❊

1. Combine yeast with 1/4 cup lukewarm water in a large mixing bowl. Add flour, 1 tsp olive oil, and 1/2 tsp salt. Mix well until blended. Add 1/3 cup water, a little at a time, until dough is smooth.

2. Turn dough out onto a lightly floured work surface. Knead dough until it is smooth and elastic (5–10 minutes). Oil another large bowl with 1 tsp olive oil. Place dough in bowl, and turn to coat. Cover with a towel, and let rise in a warm place for 1 hour or until doubled in size.

3. Preheat oven to 350°F. Line two cookie sheets with parchment paper or grease with oil. Take dough out of the bowl, and place on a lightly floured work surface. Lightly dust the top of the dough and a rolling pin with flour. Roll out the dough to about 1/8-inch thickness. Cut out 24 (3-inch) circles from the dough (the floured rim of a glass works fine).

1	Tbsp active dry yeast
1/4	cup lukewarm water, plus extra to smooth dough
2	cups unbleached, all-purpose flour
2	Tbsp + 2 tsp extra-virgin olive oil, divided
3/4	tsp salt, divided
1	cup frozen chopped spinach, thawed and drained well
1	grated medium onion, drained well
	Juice of 1 lemon
2	Tbsp fresh mint, chopped

4. Make the filling by combining spinach, onion, lemon juice, mint, 2 Tbsp olive oil, and 1/4 tsp salt in a medium bowl. Stir well to incorporate.

5. Fill each dough circle with 1 scant teaspoon of filling. Fill a small bowl with water and keep it next to the dough. Dip your fingers into the water. Wet the outer edges of the dough circles. Fold the bottom half of the circle up to the middle. Pinch in the top two sides of the circle to form a triangle. If the dough does not seal easily, use more water to coat the edges. Repeat with remaining dough circles.

6. Place 12 triangles on each cookie sheet, leaving space between them. Bake for 20–30 minutes, until golden brown, making sure not to open the oven during the first 10 minutes of baking. Serve warm. (Tip: If you're making these in advance, let cool, place in an airtight container, and freeze for up to a month.)

Healthy Living Tradition

Bread filled with vegetables makes a perfect portable snack. Make extras, and freeze them. Bring them along on car trips or for light snacks.

Exchanges/Choices		Calories	65	Sodium	80mg
1/2 Starch		Calories from Fat	15	**Total Carbohydrate**	10g
1/2 Fat		**Total Fat**	1.5g	Dietary Fiber	1g
		Saturated Fat	0.2g	Sugars	1g
Serves 24		Trans Fat	0.0g	**Protein**	2g
Serving Size: 1 triangle		**Cholesterol**	0mg		

This ubiquitous Provençal street food combines the region's French and Italian influences with local specialties. Try serving *pissaladiere* as an appetizer at a casual party or buffet, or enjoy it with salad for a light dinner. A baking stone and dough scraper are helpful when making this recipe. If you don't have them, use high-quality baking sheets and a sharp knife. Parchment paper and a pizza peel are also required.

Classic Provençal Olive, Anchovy, and Onion Pizza

❋ Pissaladiere ❋

1. Place the yeast and 1 tsp salt in a small bowl, and add 1/2 cup warm (110°F) water. Stir. Let stand for 10 minutes.

2. Place flour in a large bowl, and stir in yeast mixture, 1 Tbsp olive oil, and 1/2 cup warm water. Stir to combine until dough forms a ball.

3. Lightly flour a work surface and your hands, and transfer ball to work surface. Knead the dough gently for 5 minutes or until it feels elastic. Coat a large bowl with 1 Tbsp olive oil. Place the dough in the bowl, and turn to coat. Cover tightly with plastic wrap, and place in a draft-free area. Let rise until doubled in size, about 1 1/2 hours, or place in the refrigerator for 16–24 hours.

1	tsp rapid-rise instant yeast
1 1/2	tsp kosher or French sea salt, divided
2	cups bread flour, plus extra for work surface
6 1/2	Tbsp extra-virgin olive oil, divided
1 3/4	lb yellow onions, sliced thinly
3	cloves garlic, minced
	Pinch freshly ground black pepper
1/2	cup niçoise olives, pitted
20	anchovy fillets, rinsed and patted dry
1	tsp Herbes de Provence (p. 277)

4. Heat 1 1/2 Tbsp olive oil in a large skillet over high heat until oil begins to release its aroma. Add onions, 1/2 tsp salt, and garlic. Cook until onions begin to brown, about 10 minutes. Reduce heat to medium low. Cook until onions have softened and are golden brown (about 15–20 minutes). Remove from heat, set aside, and let cool.

5. Preheat the oven to 500°F. Cut out two pieces of parchment paper that are the same size as your baking/ pizza stone. Place baking stone in the oven.

6. When dough has doubled, remove from bowl, and place it on a lightly floured work surface. Divide the dough in half with a sharp knife or dough scraper. Shape each piece into a ball, place the seam side down, and brush each with 1/2 Tbsp olive oil. Place plastic wrap over the top, and let rest for 10 minutes.

7. Coat your fingers and palms with 1 Tbsp olive oil. Place parchment paper on a work surface. Hold dough pieces up in the air, and gently stretch them into 12-inch rectangles. Place dough on parchment paper, and shape into 14 × 8-inch ovals. Using your fingertips, make dimples on top of the ovals. Brush dough with remaining 1 Tbsp olive oil.

8. Leaving a 1/2-inch border around the edges, sprinkle black pepper and olives over the pizzas (half on each). Arrange anchovies (10 per pizza) in an interlocking pattern down the middle of the pizzas, and sprinkle each pizza with 1/2 tsp *Herbes de Provence*. Holding the parchment paper, carefully slide pizzas onto a pizza peel and then onto the baking stones, keeping the parchment underneath. Bake 13–15 minutes or until golden brown.

9. Remove pizzas from the oven by carefully lifting parchment paper onto the pizza peel. Slide parchment out from underneath the peel. Scatter caramelized onions and garlic across the top. Cool for 5 minutes, and cut into slices.

Healthy Living Tradition

Onions are used in a wide variety of Mediterranean folk recipes. Since ancient times, they've been believed to protect from illnesses and even "the evil eye." Regardless of their medicinal virtues, flavorful onions are wonderful when used as either a base or garnish.

Exchanges/Choices				
1 1/2 Starch	Calories	235	Sodium	455mg
1 Vegetable	Calories from Fat	90	**Total Carbohydrate**	30g
2 Fat	**Total Fat**	10.0g	Dietary Fiber	2g
	Saturated Fat	1.4g	Sugars	4g
	Trans Fat	0.0g	**Protein**	6g
Serves 10 (2 pizzas)	**Cholesterol**	5mg		
Serving Size: 1/10 recipe				

Sicily, like the rest of Italy, is home to two kinds of pizza. At lunch, street stands sell *pizza a taglio* (pizza by the slice), which is formed and baked in large rectangular pans and has a thick crust that resembles flatbread. At dinner, *pizzerie* sell rounded pizzas with thin crusts. Both types are available with numerous toppings. This is a simple, traditional version that can be served as an appetizer, as a snack, or with a meal.

Sicilian Pizza with Olives, Tomatoes, and Oregano

❋ *Pizza alla Siciliana* ❋

1. Dissolve yeast in 1/4 cup lukewarm water in a small bowl.

2. Pour flours into a large bowl, and make a well in the center. Add salt and remaining water. Mix well to combine. Dough should form a ball. If dough is sticky, add more flour a tablespoon at a time. Transfer to lightly floured work surface. Knead for 5–10 minutes or until dough is smooth and elastic. Shape it into a ball.

3. Coat a large bowl with 1 Tbsp olive oil. Place dough inside, and turn to coat. Cover with plastic wrap and a kitchen towel. Place in a draft-free area to rise for 1–1 1/2 hours or until doubled in size.

4. After dough has risen, knock it down, and turn it out onto a lightly floured work surface. Coat an 11 × 15-inch rectangle stone or metal baking pan with 1 Tbsp olive oil.

1	**package or 2 1/2 tsp active dry yeast**
1	**cup lukewarm water, divided**
3	**cups unbleached all-purpose flour, plus extra for work surface**
1/2	**cup unbleached bread flour**
1/2	**tsp sea salt**
3	**Tbsp extra-virgin olive oil, divided**
1 1/4	**cups boxed chopped tomatoes**
2	**tsp dried oregano**
1/2	**cup black (kalamata or Gaeta) olives, pitted and roughly chopped**
1	**can anchovies, drained, if desired**

5. Roll dough out to form an 11 × 15-inch rectangle. Transfer dough to the coated pan, and stretch to fit. Brush 1 Tbsp olive oil on top of the pizza dough, and use your fingers to make dimples across the top. Cover with foil. Let rest for 30 minutes.

6. Preheat the oven to 500°F. After the dough has rested for 30 minutes, remove foil, and cover the pizza with a thin layer of the tomatoes. Place the oregano in the palm of your hands and rub them together over the pizza to break up the oregano, release its flavor, and scatter it evenly. Arrange olives and anchovies (if using) over the pizza. Bake, uncovered, for 20–25 minutes or until golden. Remove from oven, and let cool slightly. Cut into 15 pieces, and serve.

Healthy Living Tradition

Large servings of carbohydrates can send blood glucose levels high. By having small servings of high-carbohydrate foods, like this pizza, people with diabetes can still enjoy flavorful dishes and manage their diabetes.

Exchanges/Choices	Calories	150	Sodium	125mg
1 1/2 Starch 1/2 Fat	Calories from Fat	30	**Total Carbohydrate**	26g
	Total Fat	3.5g	Dietary Fiber	1g
Serves 15	Saturated Fat	0.5g	Sugars	1g
Serving Size: 1 piece	Trans Fat	0.0g	**Protein**	4g
	Cholesterol	0mg		

When I started developing this recipe, I intended to reproduce the yeasty date-stuffed bread rings that are often eaten for breakfast in the eastern Mediterranean, the kind of food that older people love, but kids must be coaxed into eating. What I ended up with were these elegant little brioches, which look like tall muffins. These breads can be baked in advance and frozen in resealable plastic bags. To serve, defrost to room temperature and reheat for a few minutes in a preheated 350°F oven. They're great with breakfast or brunch or as a teatime treat.

Date-Stuffed Brioche Breads

1. Sprinkle yeast over water in a large bowl fitted to an electric mixer with a paddle attachment. Let stand for 5 minutes, until soft and bubbly. Add 1/4 cup warm milk, 1/2 cup oil, sugar, eggs, and salt. Mix until combined. Blend in all-purpose flour a little at a time. Blend in pastry flour a little at a time, until batter is smooth. Turn the mixer off, and scrape down the sides of the bowl. Using the dough hook, knead batter for about 5 minutes.

2. Coat a large bowl with 1 Tbsp oil, and transfer dough to it. Cover with plastic wrap, and let stand for 1 hour.

3. Make the filling by combining dates and orange blossom water in a food processor. Process to form a paste. (If mixture is crumbly or hard, add water, a tablespoon at a time, until a paste is formed.)

4 1/2 tsp active dry yeast
1/4 cup warm water
1/4 cup + 2 Tbsp warm nonfat milk
1/2 cup + 1 Tbsp canola oil, divided
1/4 cup natural sugar
   4 eggs
1/4 tsp salt
   2 cups unbleached, all-purpose flour
   2 cups whole-wheat pastry flour
1/2 lb dates, pitted
   2 tsp orange blossom water
1/4 cup sesame seeds

4. Line 15 cups of 2 1/2-inch muffin pans. After dough has risen, punch down. Spoon mixture into muffin pans, filling each 2/3 full. Using the back of a wet spoon, smooth out the tops of each muffin, and place 1 tsp date mixture in the center. Cover the date mixture with the remaining batter (by now muffin cups should be full), and smooth the tops once again. Allow muffin batter to rise for 30 minutes.

5. Preheat oven to 350°F. When batter has risen, brush the tops with 2 Tbsp milk, and scatter sesame seeds among them. Bake for 20–25 minutes or until golden. Let cool before serving.

Healthy Living Tradition

Homemade baked goods are wholesome and nutritious. An extra incentive for baking at home is that you can create unique recipes that aren't available in stores. Baking is a fun and inexpensive activity for kids, too.

Exchanges/Choices	Calories	285	Sodium	60mg
2 Starch	Calories from Fat	100	**Total Carbohydrate**	40g
1/2 Fruit	**Total Fat**	11.0g	Dietary Fiber	4g
2 Fat	Saturated Fat	1.3g	Sugars	13g
	Trans Fat	0.0g	**Protein**	6g
Serves 15	**Cholesterol**	55mg		
Serving Size: 1 roll				

Simit **are popular street snacks in Turkey.** They are sold at busy traffic intersections throughout the country. The size of the *simit* range from small, single-serving sizes (which are what this recipe makes) to large rings that are meant to be shared. They are traditionally served with tea for a snack or with jams and cheeses for breakfast. This recipe can be frozen in plastic bags for up to a month. To serve, thaw at room temperature and warm in the oven.

Mini Turkish Sesame Bread Rings

❋ **Simit** ❋

1. Preheat oven to 425°F. Coat two baking pans with extra canola oil, and set aside.

2. Sift flour and salt into a large bowl. Make a hole in the middle. Add olive oil, 3 Tbsp canola oil, 6 Tbsp water, 1/4 cup milk, and the egg. Mix well until a dough forms.

3. On a lightly floured work surface, knead dough for 5–10 minutes, until it becomes smooth and elastic. Roll the dough into a 12-inch log, and cut it into eight (1 1/2-inch-long) pieces.

4. On a work surface, use your hands to roll each piece into an 8-inch long log. Wrap the log around to form a circle, and press the ends to seal. Place rings on a baking sheet. Brush with remaining 1/4 cup milk. Sprinkle 2 tsp sesame seeds on top of each ring and bake, side by side, on the bottom rack of the oven for 20–25 minutes or until golden and crispy. Let cool and serve.

2 1/4 **cups unbleached bread flour**
1/2 **tsp salt**
2 **tsp extra-virgin olive oil**
3 **Tbsp canola oil, plus extra for greasing pans**
1/2 **cup nonfat milk, divided**
1 **egg, lightly beaten**
1/3 **cup (16 tsp) sesame seeds**

Healthy Living Tradition

Making your own homemade snacks is a great way to increase the quality of food you eat while also eliminating trans fats and chemical additives.

Exchanges/Choices	Calories	270	Sodium	165mg
2 Starch	Calories from Fat	110	Total Carbohydrate	33g
2 Fat	Total Fat	12.0g	Dietary Fiber	2g
	Saturated Fat	1.2g	Sugars	2g
Serves 8	Trans Fat	0.0g	Protein	8g
Serving Size: 1 ring	Cholesterol	25mg		

This recipe was inspired by my friend Sheilah Kaufman's recipe from *A Taste of Turkish Cuisine*, which she co-wrote with Nur Ilkin. I like to make this recipe in muffin tins and serve them with *Southern French-Style Herb-Roasted Turkey* (p. 106), *Chicken with Carrots and Leeks* (p. 97), or *Mixed Vegetable Cassoulet* (p. 132). As a snack, they also taste great covered with sugar-free preserves.

Turkish Corn Bread

1. Preheat oven to 350°F. Coat an 8-inch round cake pan or 12 cup muffin pan with 1 tsp olive oil. Combine cornmeal, salt, 1 tsp olive oil, baking powder, and sugar in a large bowl. Add the boiling water. Stir to mix until all of the water is incorporated in the mixture. Pour the cornmeal mixture into the prepared pan. Wet your hands, and press down to smooth the top.

2. *If making muffins:* Bake for 20 minutes. *If making a cake:* Bake for 10 minutes. Cover the pan with foil, and bake for 20–30 minutes more or until golden and firm.

3. Let cool slightly. Serve warm, or let cool and wrap in plastic wrap and foil to freeze.

2 tsp extra-virgin olive oil, divided
2 1/2 cups stone-ground 100% whole-grain medium-grind cornmeal
1/2 Tbsp salt
2 tsp baking powder
1 tsp sugar
2 cups boiling water

Healthy Living Tradition

An advantage of stone-ground cornmeal is that the nutritious heart of the corn germ is ground into the cornmeal itself, retaining its natural oils and vitamins.

Exchanges/Choices	Calories	100	Sodium	360mg
1 1/2 Starch	Calories from Fat	15	Total Carbohydrate	20g
	Total Fat	1.5g	Dietary Fiber	2g
Serves 12	Saturated Fat	0.3g	Sugars	0g
Serving Size: 1 muffin	Trans Fat	0.0g	Protein	2g
	Cholesterol	0mg		

Flavor Enhancers

Ingenious Herb and Spice Mixes and Secret Sauces

While fresh fruits and vegetables and grains are the staple of the Mediterranean kitchen, flavor enhancers give distinctive taste and regional appeal to the dishes of the region. By learning the techniques of combining spices, herbs, and sauces, you will learn the essence of regional Mediterranean cuisine. You'll soon have an arsenal of techniques to use whenever the occasion calls for it.

Sauces have been the base of French cuisine since 1815, when they were standardized in the book *French Cookery*, by French pastry chef Antonin Careme. Careme was the first person to classify the sauces into these categories:

- Béchamel (white)
- Veloutè (blond)
- Brown (demi-glace)
- Hollandaise (butter)
- Tomato (red)

These sauces are known as the *grandes sauces* (big sauces) or *sauces meres* (mother sauces) in French. European accounts of sauces date back to the Romans, who used sauces to enhance taste. The best sauces of the day contained so many ingredients that it was impossible for diners to determine what the recipes were. Our modern-day sauces, by contrast, contain relatively few ingredients and seek to enhance the natural flavors of the food they accompany, rather than mask them. In the regions of France along the Mediterranean coastline, olive oil and fresh herb combinations are much more common than the butter-based sauces.

In this chapter, you'll find a classic French *Herbes de Provence* (p. 277) that will transform ordinary chicken into a Mediterranean masterpiece. You'll also find the recipe for spicy *Moroccan Harissa Sauce* (p. 278), which will add zip to any meal, and creamy Middle Eastern *Tahini Sauce* (p. 279), which is both healthful and flavorful. Italian *Gremolata* (p. 280) topping is a last-minute garnish that looks great and is good for you.

This chapter also contains recipes for six essential spice mixes that add complexity of flavor to everything from dips and soups to stews and grilled meats. By keeping spice jars full of Egyptian *Baharat Spice Mix* (p. 281), Italian *Aglione* mix (p. 282), *Italian Poultry Seasoning* (p. 283), *Moroccan Ras el Hanout Spice Mix* (p. 284), *Spanish Paella Seasoning* (p. 285), and *Wild Thyme Spice Mix* (p. 286) on hand, you'll never lack inspiration in the kitchen. Adding these mixes to the most basic dishes will greatly enhance their flavor without adding calories or fat. In addition, many of the spices in the mixes contain healthful properties themselves.

Ingredients for this ubiquitous spice mixture are often found at open-air and roadside markets in Provence. Dried, locally grown herbs are mixed together, crushed, and then sold in plastic bags, colorful cloth sacks, or small clay pots. You can easily make your own version with the dried herbs you have on hand and use it to season grilled and roasted vegetables and meats.

Herbes de Provence

1. Combine herbs in a large bowl. Mix well to combine. Store in a tightly covered glass jar away from heat.

2 **Tbsp dried sage**
2 **Tbsp dried thyme**
2 **Tbsp dried marjoram**
2 **Tbsp dried basil**
2 **Tbsp fennel seeds**
2 **Tbsp dried oregano**
2 **Tbsp dried mint**
2 **Tbsp dried rosemary**
2 **Tbsp dried lavender**
2 **Tbsp dried tarragon**

Healthy Living Tradition

Allow your taste buds to determine which herbs go into your Herbes de Provence recipe. If you don't like one, simply omit it. This is the way recipes have been created for centuries in the Mediterranean.

Exchanges/Choices	Calories	10	Sodium	0mg
Free food	Calories from Fat	0	Total Carbohydrate	1g
	Total Fat	0.0g	Dietary Fiber	1g
Makes 1 1/4 cup	Saturated Fat	0.1g	Sugars	0g
Serving Size: 1 Tbsp	Trans Fat	0.0g	**Protein**	0g
	Cholesterol	0mg		

Harissa sauce is a fiery Moroccan condiment used to add flavor and heat to poultry, meats, and fish. Keep in mind that using cayenne pepper will make the sauce very hot, whereas using crushed red pepper will be milder. The sauce can be stored in an airtight container in the refrigerator for up to a month. Harissa can also be purchased bottled at Middle Eastern markets.

Moroccan Harissa Sauce

❈ Salsit Harissa ❈

1. Grind the spices, garlic, and salt together with a mortar and pestle or in a spice or coffee grinder. Just before serving, add the olive oil to the spice mixture. Place in a medium saucepan. Cook over medium heat, stirring constantly, for 5 minutes or until flavors are incorporated. Let cool, and store in a tightly sealed container in the refrigerator.

2   **Tbsp cayenne pepper or crushed red pepper**
1   **tsp fennel seeds**
1   **tsp caraway seeds**
1   **tsp ground cumin**
2   **cloves garlic, crushed**
1/2   **tsp kosher salt**
3/4   **cup extra-virgin olive oil**

Healthy Living Tradition

Caraway is one of the oldest cultivated spices in human history. Findings from Stone Age archeological sites show that early Europeans used it in cooking. It is referred to in Egyptian papyri and in Greek and Roman writings. It is still used in Egypt to suppress colic in babies.

Exchanges/Choices		Calories	10	Sodium	5mg
Free food		Calories from Fat	10	**Total Carbohydrate**	0g
		Total Fat	1.0g	Dietary Fiber	0g
Makes 3/4 cup		Saturated Fat	0.2g	Sugars	0g
Serving Size: 1/4 tsp		Trans Fat	0.0g	**Protein**	0g
		Cholesterol	0mg		

Tahini is a sesame paste made from pressing the oil from sesame seeds. The attractive flowers of the tropical sesame plant produce sesame seeds as they dry up. These flowers yield about 1 Tbsp seeds per pod. Because sesame plants are grown in abundance in the American South, its cost remains relatively low.

Tahini Sauce

1. Combine tahini, lemon juice, and vinegar in a medium bowl, mixing well. Add water, one tablespoon at a time, to thin the sauce until it reaches a syrupy consistency (about 3 Tbsp). Stir in chili powder and salt. Cover. Store in the refrigerator until needed.

1/4	cup tahini
1	tsp lemon juice
1	tsp vinegar
Dash	chili powder
1/4	tsp salt

Healthy Living Tradition

Keep extra Tahini Sauce in the refrigerator. It is a nutritious topping and sauce for many dishes.

Exchanges/Choices					
1 Fat		Calories	45	Sodium	80mg
		Calories from Fat	35	**Total Carbohydrate**	2g
		Total Fat	4.0g	Dietary Fiber	1g
Makes 8 Tbsp		Saturated Fat	0.6g	Sugars	0g
Serving Size: 1 Tbsp		Trans Fat	0.0g	**Protein**	1g
		Cholesterol	0mg		
Vegan dish					

Gremolata is a delicious blend of garlic, lemon zest, and parsley. In the U.S., it is commonly used to top *osso bucco*, braised veal shanks. It's also a wonderful topping for any soup, stew, or meat dish. In addition, when garlic and parsley are combined in equal portions, the parsley prevents the bad breath that raw garlic can cause.

Gremolata

1. Combine garlic, parsley, and lemon zest in a small bowl or jar with a lid. Stir to combine, and cover. Use immediately.

2 cloves garlic, finely chopped
2 Tbsp fresh Italian parsley, finely chopped
Grated zest of 1 lemon

Healthy Living Tradition

Parsley is common in Italian cooking. It's easy to grow parsley indoors in pots or outdoors in a garden. Try growing your own, so you'll always have it on hand.

Exchanges/Choices		Calories	10	Sodium	0mg
Free food		Calories from Fat	0	**Total Carbohydrate**	3g
		Total Fat	0.0g	Dietary Fiber	0g
Makes 1/4 cup		Saturated Fat	0.0g	Sugars	0g
Serving Size: 1/4 cup		Trans Fat	0.0g	**Protein**	0g
		Cholesterol	0mg		

Baharat **is the Arabic name given to various spice mixes throughout the Arab world.** Each country has its own basic *baharat* for fish, poultry, and meat. Homemade mixes vary according to prices, availability, and personal preference. I like to prepare it in large quantities ahead of time. That way, when I'm cooking, I don't need to take the time to find the individual spices. Feel free to alter this recipe to your tastes.

Baharat Spice Mix

1. Place all ingredients in a glass jar. Cover jar with lid, and shake to combine. Store for up to 2 months in a cool, dark place.

1/4 **cup ground black pepper**
1/8 **cup dried ground coriander**
1/8 **cup ground cloves**
2 **Tbsp ground cumin**
1/8 **cup ground cardamom**
1 **tsp fresh nutmeg**
1/4 **cup paprika**
1/8 **cup ground ginger**
Few dashes crushed red pepper

Healthy Living Tradition

Take time to discover new spice combinations and scents. Spices are a great way to add flavor without adding calories and fat. They also release wonderful aromas while cooking, which allows our sense of smell to transport us to magical locations.

Exchanges/Choices				
Free food	Calories	15	Sodium	0mg
	Calories from Fat	5	**Total Carbohydrate**	3g
	Total Fat	0.5g	Dietary Fiber	1g
Makes 1 cup	Saturated Fat	0.1g	Sugars	1g
Serving Size: 1 Tbsp	Trans Fat	0.0g	**Protein**	1g
	Cholesterol	0mg		

***Aglione* is a traditional garlic-based flavor enhancer of the Emilia Romagna region of Italy.** Home to Bologna and Parma, Emilia Romagna is known as the culinary center of Italy. Try adding this mixture to soups, stews, grilled meat, fish, poultry, and vegetables for a tasty, authentic change. Juniper berries are the female seed cones found on some juniper trees. They are what is used to flavor gin and can be found in gourmet and specialty stores.

Aglione

1. Remove the leaves from the rosemary sprigs, and discard stems. Combine rosemary, sage, garlic, and juniper berries on a chopping board. Chop finely, and place in a small bowl. Stir in pepper. Transfer to a jar with a tight-fitting lid, and store in the refrigerator for a few weeks.

2 **rosemary sprigs**
5 **fresh sage leaves**
1 **clove garlic, peeled**
1 **tsp juniper berries, crushed**
1/4 **tsp freshly ground black pepper**

Healthy Living Tradition

The ancient Greeks fed juniper berries to Olympic athletes, believing it would increase their stamina.

Exchanges/Choices				
Free food	**Calories**	5	**Sodium**	0mg
	Calories from Fat	0	**Total Carbohydrate**	1g
	Total Fat	0.0g	Dietary Fiber	0g
Makes 1/4 cup	Saturated Fat	0.0g	Sugars	1g
Serving Size: 1 Tbsp	Trans Fat	0.0g	**Protein**	0g
	Cholesterol	0mg		

Each year before the first frost, I pick my herb plants down to the roots. Next, I wash them and dry them in a closet. When the herbs are dry, I crush them to make the following mix. It tastes delicious with chicken, turkey, and duck.

Italian Poultry Seasoning

1. Combine dried rosemary, sage, thyme, and salt in a small, airtight container. Store in a cool pantry for up to 1 year.

1/4 cup dried rosemary
2 Tbsp dried sage
1 Tbsp dried thyme
1 tsp sea salt

Healthy Living Tradition

The oil extracted from thyme is called thymol. The Ancient Egyptians used thymol to preserve mummies. It is also an antiseptic that is used in mouthwashes.

Exchanges/Choices		Calories	10	Sodium	295mg
Free food		Calories from Fat	0	**Total Carbohydrate**	2g
		Total Fat	0.0g	Dietary Fiber	1g
Makes 1/2 cup		Saturated Fat	0.2g	Sugars	0g
Serving Size: 1 Tbsp		Trans Fat	0.0g	**Protein**	0g
		Cholesterol	0mg		

Ras el hanout **means "head of the shop" in Arabic.** Some versions of this spice mix contain up to 27 different ingredients. Spice mixes are an integral part of Moroccan cuisine, and many people, as well as spice vendors, claim that their version is best.

Moroccan Ras el Hanout Spice Mix

1. Pour all ingredients into a bowl, and stir until combined. Place in an airtight container inside a cupboard, away from heat, for up to 1 month.

2 tsp ground cumin
2 tsp ground ginger
3 tsp kosher or sea salt
2 tsp freshly ground black pepper
1 1/2 tsp ground cinnamon
1 tsp ground coriander
1 tsp cayenne
1 tsp allspice
1 tsp saffron

Healthy Living Tradition

All across North Africa, spices are used to prevent illnesses and maintain healthy body functions. Take the time to research which foods are appropriate for your body type and to add new flavors to your meals.

Exchanges/Choices			
Free food	Calories	0	Sodium	120mg
	Calories from Fat	0	Total Carbohydrate	0g
	Total Fat	0.0g	Dietary Fiber	0g
Makes 1/4 cup	Saturated Fat	0.0g	Sugars	0g
Serving Size: 1/4 tsp	Trans Fat	0.0g	Protein	0g
	Cholesterol	0mg		

Keep this delicious mixture on hand for making paella or sprinkling on fried potatoes, seafood, and vegetables. Store this spice mix, along with other red spices, in airtight containers in the refrigerator to retain maximum flavor.

Spanish Paella Seasoning

1. Combine ingredients in a small airtight container, and store in the refrigerator for up to 1 year.

1/4	cup sweet paprika
1	tsp high-quality saffron
1/4	tsp crushed red chili pepper
1	Tbsp salt

Healthy Living Tradition

The world's most expensive spice, saffron, is cultivated from the stigmas of the crocus flower in the autumn. Its English name is derived from the plural of the feminine form of the Arabic word for "yellow," saffra. Saffron provides a bright yellow pigment and gives unique flavor to drinks, savories, and sweets.

Exchanges/Choices	Calories	5	Sodium	435mg
Free food	Calories from Fat	0	Total Carbohydrate	1g
	Total Fat	0.0g	Dietary Fiber	0g
Makes 1/3 cup	Saturated Fat	0.0g	Sugars	1g
Serving Size: 1 tsp	Trans Fat	0.0g	Protein	0g
	Cholesterol	0mg		

Za'taar is the name of both wild thyme and a spice mix made with wild thyme in the Middle East. Particularly popular in Lebanon, *za'taar* is great for sprinkling on pita chips, yogurt cheese, breads, and plain pizza dough. Some people like to dip fresh, hot pita bread in olive oil and then in *za'taar*.

Wild Thyme Spice Mix

❋ Za'taar ❋

1. Combine ingredients in an airtight container. Shake well to combine, seal, and store in a dark, cool place for up to 1 year.

1/4 cup dried ground za'taar (wild thyme) or regular dried thyme
1/4 cup dried ground coriander
1/4 cup sesame seeds
1 Tbsp dried ground cumin
1 Tbsp anise seeds
1 Tbsp fennel seeds
1 Tbsp sea salt

Healthy Living Tradition

Coriander is made from dried cilantro seeds. It imparts a sweet and spicy flavor to savory dishes.

Exchanges/Choices	Calories	5	Sodium	150mg
Free food	Calories from Fat	0	**Total Carbohydrate**	1g
	Total Fat	0.0g	Dietary Fiber	0g
Makes 1 cup	Saturated Fat	0.1g	Sugars	0g
Serving Size: 1 tsp	Trans Fat	0.0g	**Protein**	0g
	Cholesterol	0mg		

This unique Egyptian seafood seasoning is a great alternative to high-sodium commercial varieties.

Seafood Seasoning

1. Combine ingredients in a small airtight container, and store in the refrigerator for up to 1 year.

1 tsp cumin
1 tsp turmeric
1 tsp allspice
1 tsp coriander

Healthy Living Tradition

Turmeric has a notable role in history. It has been used to repel ants in gardens, as a natural dye, and as an antiseptic and anti-inflammatory agent in traditional medicine since antiquity.

Exchanges/Choices				
Free food				
	Calories	5	**Sodium**	0mg
	Calories from Fat	0	**Total Carbohydrate**	1g
	Total Fat	0.0g	Dietary Fiber	0g
Makes 4 tsp	Saturated Fat	0.0g	Sugars	0g
Serving Size: 1 tsp	Trans Fat	0.0g	**Protein**	0g
	Cholesterol	0mg		

Index

Vegetables, Other

Recipes by Origin

Other Titles from the American Diabetes Association

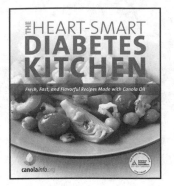 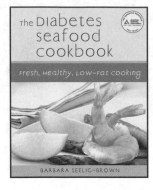 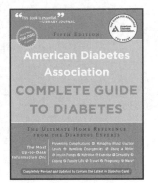 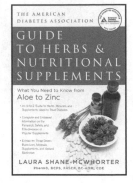

The Heart-Smart Diabetes Kitchen:
Fresh, Fast, and Flavorful Recipes Made with Canola Oil
by the American Diabetes Association and CanolaInfo
Bring the taste of fresh, natural ingredients and wholesome meals to your table. Featuring over 150 recipes made with canola oil, this cookbook allows you to serve dishes that are low in saturated fat and cholesterol but high in flavor in no time. It's just what the doctor, and your inner chef, ordered.
Order no. 4677-01; Price $18.95

The Diabetes Seafood Cookbook
by Barbara Seelig-Brown
Seafood is the perfect choice for anyone looking to eat healthfully without skimping on flavor. From freshwater and saltwater fish to crab, shrimp, and clams, this book delivers over 150 delicious recipes for the perfect party appetizer, a delightful family dinner, or a satisfying side dish.
Order no. 4670.01; Price $18.95

American Diabetes Association Complete Guide to Diabetes, 5th Edition
by American Diabetes Association
Have all the tips and information on diabetes that you need close at hand. The world's largest collection of diabetes self-care tips, techniques, and tricks for solving diabetes-related problems is back in its fifth edition, and it's bigger and better than ever before.
Order no. 4809-05; Price $22.95

American Diabetes Association Guide to Herbs & Nutritional Supplements:
What You Need to Know from Aloe to Zinc
by Laura Shane-McWhorter, PharmD, BCPS, FASCP, BC-ADM, CDE
Get reliable, unbiased information on nutritional supplements, herbs, and other natural products. This book covers everything you need to know about 40 of the most popular alternative therapies used for diabetes, including cinnamon, garlic, ginseng, magnesium, and more! Before taking anything that may have a profound effect on your health, know what you're taking.
Order no. 4889-01; Price 16.95

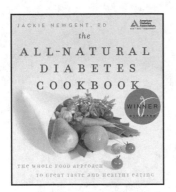 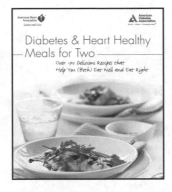 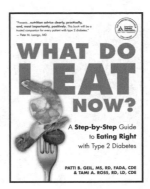 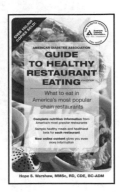

The All-Natural Diabetes Cookbook:
The Whole Food Approach to Great Taste and Healthy Eating
by Jackie Newgent, RD
Instead of relying on artificial sweeteners or not-so-real substitutions to reduce calories, sugar, and fat,
The All-Natural Diabetes Cookbook takes a different approach, focusing on naturally delicious fresh foods
and whole-food ingredients to create fantastic meals that deliver amazing taste and well-rounded nutrition.
And absolutely nothing is artificial.
Order no. 4663-01; Price $18.95

Diabetes & Heart Healthy Meals for Two
by the American Diabetes Association and the American Heart Association
If you or a loved one has diabetes, you need to eat heart-healthy meals. The simple, flavorful recipes were
designed for those looking to improve or maintain their cardiovascular health. Each recipe is for two people,
making this book perfect for adults without children in the house or for those who want to keep leftovers to
a minimum. With over 170 recipes, there are countless options to keep you heart at its healthiest and your
blood glucose under control.
Order no. 4673-01; Price $18.95

What Do I Eat Now? A Step-by-Step Guide to Eating Right with Type 2 Diabetes
by Patti B. Geil, MS, RD, FADA, CDE, and Tami A. Ross, RD, LD, CDE
You've been told to eat healthy, but what does that mean? With this book, you'll know exactly what it means. In
only 4 weeks, you will learn how to eat better, improve diabetes management, and live a healthier lifestyle.
Order no. 4886-01; Price $17.95

Guide to Healthy Restaurant Eating, 4th Edition
by Hope S. Warshaw, MMSc, RD, CDE, BC-ADM
Eat out without guilt or sacrifice! Newly updated, this bestselling guide features more than 7,000 menu items
for over 50 restaurant chains, with a new online database with even more content. This
is the most comprehensive guide to restaurant nutrition for people with diabetes who like to eat out.
Order no. 4819-04; Price $17.95

To order these and other great American Diabetes Association titles,
call **1-800-232-6733** or visit **http://store.diabetes.org**.
American Diabetes Association titles are also available in bookstores nationwide.